This special edition copy of *Selections
from Overcoming Hypertension* is provided to you as a service by your physician
and Searle.

It offers suggestions on diet and exercise to help you work with your doctor to
control your high blood pressure. Your
doctor will want you to follow specific
directions concerning diet, exercise, and
medicines that are appropriate for your
individual needs. Be sure to check with
your doctor before beginning a special diet
or exercise program.

We hope that you find this book
helpful.

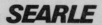

SEARLE

Dr. Kenneth H. Cooper's
Preventive Medicine Program

Selections From
Overcoming
Hypertension

Kenneth H. Cooper,
M.D., M.P.H.

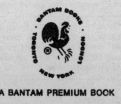

A BANTAM PREMIUM BOOK

Selections From
OVERCOMING HYPERTENSION
A Bantam Nonfiction Book
Bantam hardcover edition / March 1990
Bantam paperback edition / May 1991

Contents

1. The Much Misunderstood Challenge of Hypertension 1

2. Demystifying Those Blood Pressure Measurements 13

3. Control Through Exercise 31

4. Control Through Diet 75

5. Watch the Way You Respond—and Learn to Relax! 188

6. A Future Without Hypertension? 197

   References 200

   Appendix I 206

   Appendix II 218

   Appendix III 225

   Appendix IV 235

1

The Much Misunderstood Challenge of Hypertension

Hypertension is an illness of civilization.

Personal and professional stress, poor diet, lack of exercise—these and related features of our so-called advanced societies contribute heavily to the problems of the nearly 60 million Americans who have some form of high blood pressure.

There's a danger that as we progress toward the twenty-first century and life in our cities and suburbs becomes more pressure-ridden and unlivable, the number of those at risk for hypertension will rise. But I'm convinced that this danger can be confronted and conquered—*if*, through extensive public education, we can explain the paradoxes and perplexities of hypertension.

Hypertension is, indeed, a disease fraught with misunderstanding and confusion. For example, there's the question of just how to evaluate the danger of high blood pressure. Without doubt, in many respects hypertension poses one of the most serious threats to our health. The disease is *the* major risk factor for all forms of stroke; furthermore, it can lead to kidney failure or other serious disorders.

Paradoxically, as dangerous as this disease is, one or

even several high blood pressure readings are nothing to panic about. To be sure, hypertension is a silent killer, and the first major symptom may be death. But with an early diagnosis, you have time on your side because it typically takes ten to twenty years for hypertension to cause real damage to your health.

Furthermore, for most people with hypertension, the initial approach to treatment doesn't have to turn one's life upside down. The first line of attack usually consists of nondrug treatments rather than medication.

If you are among the 60 million Americans who now confront hypertension, here are some facts you should know:

- Your chances of controlling mild hypertension without drugs are *very good*.

- A single high reading in your doctor's office is *not* conclusive evidence of the disease.

- Your blood pressure readings may vary considerably during any given day—and those ups and downs may be quite normal.

- It's common for many people, with hypertension or without, to have two upward "bursts" of blood pressure in the morning—one immediately on awakening, and another on getting out of bed and walking about.

- Vigorous exertion (especially the type that tenses the muscles), the experience of stress or anxiety, the ingestion of caffeine, smoking, a full bladder, or simply eating immediately before a blood pressure reading is taken *may* lead to an invalid measurement.

- Excessive use of alcohol may lead to elevated blood pressure, but, paradoxically, moderate use has been linked to a lower incidence of coronary disease.

- Your *average* blood pressure (i.e., the average of multiple readings taken over one to two months, rather than one isolated reading) is the key to diagnosing hypertension.

- Many cases of hypertension have a genetic factor: In other words, there's an inherited tendency toward high blood pressure in some people. However, your genes need not be decisive! Changes in lifestyle or the administration of appropriate medications can often offset the influence of heredity.

The main focus of this book is on managing hypertension without drugs. But there are many healthy people who exercise regularly and eat correctly, yet who *can't* control their hypertension through a drug-free regimen.

We live in a high-pressure society that requires millions of those with hypertension to rely both on nondrug treatments *and* on medication. Furthermore, as the following story demonstrates, a patient can have a lot of input into the way his illness is treated.

How One Patient Participated in Choosing His Treatments

William, a busy executive in his early fifties, had been coming in for regular annual medical exams for several years, and the first few times his blood pressure had been normal.

His initial measurement, which was performed as part of a checkup for health insurance, was 130/82 (the meaning of these numbers will be explained in upcoming chapters)—well below the generally accepted "mild" or "borderline" hypertension level that begins at 140/90. During this exam I had followed the classic procedure for taking a first blood pressure, which involved the following steps:

I took several separate readings during that first visit to find how William's blood pressure responded under different circumstances. First of all, using the traditional measuring device called the sphygmomanometer, I checked his right arm while he was sitting in a chair.

The sphygmomanometer is a cufflike inflatable bladder, usually measuring 12 by 23 centimeters, which the doctor or technician wraps around the patient's upper arm and then blows up with a small hand-held bulb pump. The pressure created by the inflation of the cuff cuts off the circulation momentarily. Then, as the pressure is released, the physician listens through attached earphones for the first and last sounds of blood rushing back through the arm to determine the upper (systolic) and lower (diastolic) blood pressure readings.

Before taking the pressure, I made sure that William had been seated for at least five minutes and was leaning back in a relaxed position. His right arm, on which I had placed the sphygmomanometer, was supported at about heart level by the arm of the chair.

Then I checked his left arm and found the pressure to be the same as on the right. (Sometimes the pressures in the arms are different, and in such situations we go with the arm that has the higher reading.) Next, I took his pressure lying down on his back and also standing up. As with many people, his standing pressure was somewhat higher than in the other positions.

Finally, to get his true pressure, I took two more readings while he was in the sitting position with the cuff on his right arm. By figuring the average of the three sitting measurements of his right arm, I was able to establish his true blood pressure during that office visit.

As is the case with many patients, William had a higher reading on the first of his sitting measurements than on the two later ones. Specifically, his first measurement was 138/88, which placed him near the mild or borderline hypertensive category.

But this was a normal reaction, since many patients are under greater stress during the first phase of a medical exam than later, when the procedures and atmosphere have become more familiar. And remember the final result: His *average* blood pressure, using all three readings, was 135/80. As William's response suggests, it's important for a physician to take several readings and find the average, rather than just to go with one initial measurement, which may be unusually high. (Another option is to take three measurements, discard the first, and average the last two.)

During the next three years, as William came in for annual physicals, his blood pressure began to creep up. The second year I checked him, his average reading was 134/85; the third year, it was up to 137/88.

Clearly, there was an upward trend. Already he had almost reached the "mild" hypertension category, which begins with a diastolic reading of 90. Furthermore, he was almost up to the "borderline" systolic hypertension level, which begins at 140. In light of these developments, I wanted to be sure that William was doing everything in his power, within normal limits, to control his blood pressure.

As I questioned him, he confirmed that he was still following these instructions for preparation before his exam:

- He urinated before the test (a full bladder will increase pressure).

- He refrained from eating or ingesting caffeine for at least sixty minutes before the test.

- He avoided vigorous exercise just before the measurements were taken.

Also, I knew William wasn't on any drugs, such as steroids, which might raise his blood pressure. Nor was he a smoker or overweight. Furthermore, he had gone on a low-fat diet as part of a personal health program, and he regularly ran about ten miles a week. All these are part of the plan recommended for preventing and controlling hypertension.

But William's pressure still was rising, and I was determined to head it off. I recommended that he adjust his diet further by going on a stricter low-salt regimen. He had been watching his salt consumption, but not very closely. I estimated that he was eating fewer than 4 grams of sodium a day, or somewhat below the national average of 4 to 6 grams daily. But a more severe diet averaging about 2 grams of sodium a day (which works out to about 5 grams of salt) seemed in order. Eager to do all he could to prevent the onset of full-blown hypertension, he agreed to try my suggestions.

In addition, because William was under relatively heavy pressure at work, I recommended that he try some relaxation techniques to reduce his stress level. Again, he said he'd try.

But when he returned in three months for a progress evaluation, the situation was worse. His average blood pressure readings had risen to 145/95. These measurements put him well up into the mild hypertension category on his diastolic (lower) blood pressure number, and the borderline classification on his systolic (upper) pressure.

The nondrug treatments we had tried so far hadn't succeeded in controlling the upward march—so what was the next step?

First, it was necessary to establish a firm diagnosis of hypertension so that I'd have a solid basis for prescribing further treatment. To do this, I followed a well-accepted procedure: I took several sets of average readings over the next month and came up with the same result—an average blood pressure of 145/95.

Because William's pressure had only recently moved into the mild or borderline range, I knew we had time to work on the problem. Typically, it may take ten to twenty years before hypertension does any serious damage to the body, and William certainly hadn't had his condition that long. So, knowing that stress was most likely a part of his problem, I decided to try another nondrug approach.

"I know your job is a pressure cooker," I said. "Any way you can change that?"

"I can't quit—this is my life!" he said.

"I realize that. But what *can* you do to reduce the stress you're under at work?"

He thought about it and decided to cut back on his work load and spend more time unwinding with his family in the evenings and on weekends.

I also recommended some sources for learning relaxation techniques, including several books on the subject and also a psychologist who specialized in that area. Some people who practice these methods regularly—and at the same time follow sound antihypertensive health practices, such as a low-salt, low-fat diet, moderate alcohol intake, and regular exercise—have lowered *both* their upper and lower blood pressure readings by 20 points or more.

William agreed to this strategy. But I wanted to know how it was working under real-life conditions, to see how particular lifestyle changes and relaxation techniques succeeded or failed *in practice* in lowering his blood pressure.

Obviously, I couldn't follow William around all day and check his blood pressure under different conditions. So I recommended that he buy a home monitoring device—which can be purchased for less than $60—and take his own blood pressure several times a day. These devices look much like the ones in your physician's office, but they're more compact and simpler to use. For example, many have digital displays, rather than a traditional clock-like dial and pointer, to show the blood pressure measurement.

After I had shown William how to take his own pressure, we identified several points during his day t' would provide a complete picture of his condition. Spec ically, he took his pressure (1) when he first got up in the morning; (2) just after he arrived at work; (3) in the midafternoon, when his job pressures were at a peak; and (4) in the evening after dinner, when he was feeling relaxed.

Over the course of a couple of weeks, William's self-recorded readings at these four times averaged out this way:

- First thing in the morning: 135/88
- Arrival at work: 140/92
- Midafternoon: 155/96
- Evening at home: 130/85

By doing this self-monitoring, William provided me with information I could not otherwise have obtained. It was evident from these readings that his blood pressure was quite normal when he was at home, away from the stresses of work. That confirmed my belief that the more time he could spend in the company of his family, the better.

Also, I suspected that his measurements were even lower while he was asleep, as most people tend to have their lowest readings at that time. To check this out, I had William take his pressure a few times when he woke up in the middle of the night. The readings were indeed lower on those occasions than they were after he awakened in the morning.

Blood pressure typically jumps up on awakening, sometimes by as much as 20 points for both the upper and lower readings. There's still another surge upward when the person gets out of bed and begins to walk about. William's total increase in pressure at these times was more on the order of about 10 points for both the systolic and diastolic readings. But he still remained in the normal range during the early morning hours.

However, William was apparently in a mild or borderline hypertensive state throughout his workday. I knew that these higher readings over a period of several hours each day could eventually lead to a permanent hypertensive condition. So I encouraged him to continue to work at reducing his stress.

Unfortunately, he couldn't do anything to bring down his blood pressure levels at work; he said that the demands on him were just too great. Furthermore, as disciplined as he was in other areas of his life, he wasn't able to stay with a regular relaxation program. Typically, these programs require participants to do meditative and breathing exercises twice a day for twenty minutes at each session, day in and day out. Some people take to such a program quite naturally, while others, perhaps because they have doubts about whether it will really work, are unable to get started.

"I just can't find the time for that," William said. "My schedule is already too packed to make time for such things. Besides, I'm just not a natural meditator."

After about six months of monitoring and consultation, William's average readings held at about 148/95. As a result, I prescribed an antihypertensive medication—one of the beta-blocker drugs, metoprolol (Lopressor).

Beta blockers are designed to lower the blood pressure by reducing the pumping action and blood output of the heart. This type of drug isn't usually appropriate for young athletes because it limits the intensity of the physical activity in which a person can engage. But the medication was fine for William because his only exercise was moderate jogging.

Fortunately, too, the possible side effects of beta blockers—which may include such reactions as fatigue, insomnia, or impotence—didn't materialize.

The end result in William's case: His blood pressure on the medication decreased to an average of 129/84—well within normal limits both in the doctor's office and in various stressful situations at work.

The Power of Cooperation

William's experience is instructive in a number of ways—especially as it shows us the value and power of cooperation between the physician and patient in dealing with hypertension.

Obviously, the initial examination and recommendation in this situation had to be made by me—the physician. But by learning to monitor his own blood pressure, both at home and at work, William contributed significantly to the process. He provided information that helped in proving the diagnosis of hypertension and in providing the groundwork for its treatment.

Two important principles underlie this need for cooperation between the hypertensive patient and the physician:

1. Your doctor needs to know your average blood pressure in order to make a definite diagnosis of hypertension. Under his guidance, you can help him gather

important information as you monitor your pressure at home and at work.

2. Your doctor's ability to make an accurate diagnosis can also be enhanced if he understands how your pressure responds in a variety of daily circumstances, whether at home, at work, or in other activities. If you experience regular, relatively high peaks of high blood pressure at work—or if your blood pressure stays up at hypertensive levels in other circumstances for sustained periods—that characteristic will place you at greater risk for permanent hypertension.

To identify those peaks and rises, *you* must learn to check your own pressure. Your doctor can't be with you to check you at those moments.

What if your doctor doesn't want this sort of help from you? He *should* welcome your willingness to cooperate with him—even if he recommends that in your case self-monitoring isn't really necessary. If he doesn't appreciate your interest, perhaps you should consider finding another physician.

In the following pages, we'll consider in great detail topics that often lend themselves to your collaboration with your physician in preventing, controlling, and curing hypertension. You'll learn:

- Ways to evaluate your risk for hypertension

- An explanation of how other coronary risk factors—such as high cholesterol, cigarette smoking, obesity, or failure to manage stress well—can actually *multiply* your risk level

- Your personal blood pressure classification

- What your blood pressure readings really mean

- The implications of "high," "low," and "normal" readings

- How to take your own blood pressure

- Why many people experience a marked increase in

blood pressure when they're tested in the doctor's office—even though they may not be hypertensive

- How exercise can reduce your blood pressure (To show you step by step how this works, I've included a complete antihypertensive aerobics program.)

- Why weight training may be dangerous if you have high blood pressure

- The levels of blood pressure that make any exercise unsafe

- A special formula to enable those on beta-blocker drugs to find their target heart rate during exercise (You'll recall that beta blockers slow down the heart rate; so those on these drugs must expect to exercise at a lower level of intensity than other athletes.)

- Why older people don't have to settle for relatively high blood pressure readings
    There's an old rule of thumb that says, "Your systolic (upper) blood pressure reading should be no higher than 100 plus your age." Using this approach, many doctors still believe that a reading of 170/90 is quite acceptable for those 70 years of age or older. Yet, I've discovered that exercise and a healthy diet and lifestyle can keep the average person's blood pressure near the levels of youth.
    In one series of studies at the Aerobics Center, for instance, the median blood pressure for those who were 60 years of age and older was 132/82—a level that would make most 30-year-olds quite happy!

- The healthy levels of blood pressure for children of all ages

- How "salt-sensitive" people can control hypertension through their diets
    There is evidence that some people, but not all, are salt-sensitive. This means that their blood

pressure tends to rise when they increase the amount of salt in their diets. By experimenting with your diet and watching the results as you monitor your blood pressure, your physician may be able to determine whether your pressure reacts negatively to salt.

Our expert nutritionists have designed menus and recipes containing an average of about 2 grams of sodium per day—a good target for those who are trying to control their salt intake. In addition, consideration has been paid to other nutritional factors that may influence blood pressure, such as fats, calcium, magnesium, potassium, and fiber. Also, lists of the sodium and other nutritional contents of various foods have been included to help you follow a low-salt diet.

- How particular foods, like licorice, may raise blood pressure levels significantly in some people

- Relaxation techniques that have proven effective in lowering blood pressure in some patients

- Ways to organize your schedule so that you can deal more successfully with the pressures of our increasingly stressful society

- The alcohol question—specifically, how much is too much?

    Research on hypertension has established that excessive consumption of alcohol may contribute to elevated blood pressure. But how much is too much? Most experts agree that "moderate" drinking is all right—but what constitutes moderation? Also, are there people whose blood pressure is "alcohol-sensitive" to the extent that they shouldn't drink at all?

2

Demystifying Those Blood Pressure Measurements

Your *true* blood pressure isn't simply one constant set of figures that a doctor can determine with one measurement once a year. Rather, blood pressure readings may vary from hour to hour—or even within a matter of minutes.

Consider a few of the possibilities:

- Many people experience large short-term jumps in blood pressure—up to 30 or 40 points, or even more—as a result of occupational or personal stresses during a typical day. One man I know underwent a 40-point increase after being pricked on the buttocks with a needle!

- The blood pressure of some patients rises much higher due to the "white-coat" phenomenon (or the "cuff syndrome," as it's sometimes called). This reaction refers to the tendency of blood pressure to rise when the person is examined by a physician or in a medical setting.

- Some weight lifters have had an increase in blood pressure to as high as 350/150 during heavy lifting.

- One 75-year-old man, whose pressure was, for his age, a very normal and healthy 120/80 at rest, went to an unusually high 270/100 during exercise on a treadmill.

Usually, 240/120 is the maximum safe ceiling for a blood pressure rise during maximal aerobic exercise. But in this case, the person consistently experienced this dramatic rise during closely monitored stress tests and then returned to normal—without any ill effects.

What are we to make of these extreme variations in blood pressure? Are they "normal" or "safe"? What is the real meaning of those two mysterious figures that are supposed to reflect our blood pressure?

In fact, all of these extremes in blood pressure may be quite safe and normal. Blood pressure is a very individual matter, and the meaning of *your* particular reading must be determined by your doctor, working cooperatively with you. To facilitate your collaboration with your physician, let's now go into more detail about the possible meanings of your personal measurements.

The Meaning of
the Measurements

When you have your blood pressure taken, you'll receive the results in the form of two numbers separated by a slash, such as 120/80. This measurement, by the way, should be read "one-twenty over eighty."

In this case, the first, or upper, number, 120, is known as the *systolic* blood pressure. This systolic figure reflects the force that's exerted against the vessel walls as the blood is pumped during the contracting or beating action of the heart. The second, or lower, number, 80, is the *diastolic* blood pressure. This diastolic reading refers to the pressure level that occurs in your vessels between heartbeats, when the heart muscle is relaxed. Both numbers are expressed in terms of "millimeters of mercury," or mm Hg, because a column of liquid mercury is used in standard sphygmomanometers to measure blood pressure.

Now, about the meanings of these figures for individual patients:

As a basic guideline, blood pressure that is below 140/90 is generally considered normal. But when readings move above 140/90, treatment of some sort, either through diet and lifestyle changes or through doctor-prescribed medications, must be considered.

In my practice, I emphasize nondrug therapies—such as exercise, weight loss, adjustment of diet, and stress-lowering strategies—for systolic blood pressures that range up to 159 and for diastolic blood pressures that range up to 94. These pressures are considered in the borderline or low-mild area of hypertension and may reflect situations where hypertension hasn't yet fully taken hold in a person's life. In these cases, a serious effort to change one's lifestyle can often reverse the progression of high blood pressure.

But pressures that are consistently 160/95 or above (and that means either the systolic *or* the diastolic at these levels) frequently signal the existence of a relatively permanent state of hypertension. In these cases, medications will usually be required in addition to nondrug treatments.

I find that remembering these simple cut-off points can often help patients remember the probable meaning of their blood pressure measurements. Still, there are many other, more detailed, specific schemes for interpreting blood pressure than the shorthand standards I've just suggested. "The 1988 Report of the Fourth Joint National Committee on Detection, Evaluation, and Treatment of High Blood Pressure," for instance, recommends these more extensive classifications and follow-up procedures:

Classification of Blood Pressure in Adults 18 Years of Age or Older

Blood Pressure Range mm Hg (mercury)	Category	Follow-up by physician
1. Diastolic blood pressure:		
<85	Normal	Recheck within 2 years
85–89	High normal	Recheck within 1 year
90–104	Mild hypertension	Confirm within 2 months
105–114	Moderate hypertension	Evaluate or refer promptly to source of care within 2 weeks
>115	Severe hypertension	Evaluate or refer immediately to source of care
2. Systolic blood pressure, when diastolic is less than 90 mm Hg:		
<140	Normal	Recheck within 2 years
140–159	Borderline isolated systolic hypertension	
>160	Isolated systolic hypertension	If systolic is in 140–199 range, confirm within 2 months. If at or above 200, evaluate or refer promptly to source of care within 2 weeks.

The Joint National Committee report also includes these explanatory notes for the above classifications, which I've edited somewhat:

Note 1. The classifications are based on the average of two or more readings on two or more occasions.

Note 2. A classification of borderline isolated systolic hypertension (i.e., systolic of 140 to 159 mm Hg) or of isolated systolic hypertension (systolic at or greater than 160) takes precedence over high-normal blood pressure (diastolic of 85 to 89) for purposes of treatment when both occur in the same person.

Note 3. If recommendations for follow-up of diastolic and systolic blood pressure are different, the shorter recommended time for rechecking and referral takes precedence.

Many physicians—including my special consultant for this book, Dr. Norman Kaplan of the University of Texas Southwestern Medical Center at Dallas, who was a member of the Joint National Committee—accept these classifications as their basic standard.

Like all definitions of hypertension, however, these Joint National Committee figures aren't written in stone. The operative classifications were different as recently as 1980, when the World Health Organization (WHO) recommended that hypertension begin at readings of 160/95.

But more recent studies have demonstrated that serious health risks may accompany even borderline hypertension, down to the lower level of 140/90. So the 1984 Third Joint National Committee elected to begin the designation of hypertension at that lower level.

Before 1984, there were obviously far fewer people who were diagnosed as hypertensive, because the blood pressure levels defining the disease were higher. Under the old 160/95 standard, for instance, 30 million Americans would be classified today as hypertensive, as compared with about 58 to 60 million under the new 140/90 standards. As might be expected, with the more stringent current definitions, doctors today are more likely to begin some sort of treatment at an earlier point than they did in the past.

Will the latest Joint National Committee recommendations on classifying and treating hypertension hold up?

If past history is any indication, they probably won't. The study of hypertension is constantly bringing new information to light, such as the value of exercise and stress-reduction techniques in treating mild hypertension. With this new information, the approaches to treatment and the meanings of various blood pressure levels are subject to constant review and change.

Even today, individual doctors who support the Joint National Committee may still "adjust" or "interpret" these figures according to the special situations faced by persons and groups they treat.

For one thing, informed doctors may be aware that one or more of a particular patient's blood pressure readings are *similar* to those characteristic of certain classifications of people. But that doesn't mean the physician will necessarily treat that patient according to the classification.

A case in point: A number of my patients are subject to the so-called white coat phenomenon, which causes both their systolic and diastolic blood pressure to shoot up 30 or more points when they come into my office for an exam. The mere stress of the visit raises their readings through the roof—even when I take their pressure several times in an effort to get an average reading.

If I chose rigidly to classify these people according to the Joint Committee's criteria, I'd be treating many of them for severe hypertension. But I've learned over the course of several exams that these people aren't really hypertensive. They just have high readings when they're in my office, and then their pressure returns to normal when they leave.

To determine their out-of-the-office readings, I've had a number of them take their own blood pressure through the use of home monitoring devices (which we'll discuss later in this chapter). Then, upon ascertaining that their elevated pressure is due to the surroundings of the medical exam, I'm in a position to classify them, and, if necessary, treat them, differently than I could if I relied only on the measurements taken in my office.

What lesson should we learn from such practical experience? Just this: Classifications such as those suggested by the Joint National Committee are essential to follow as basic guidelines. But the specific treatment, if any, for your blood pressure is a matter for your doctor, working closely with you, to decide.

Even Dr. Kaplan takes a flexible approach to the classifications. He questions, for example, whether everyone whose diastolic (lower) number is in the 85 to 89 range

should be labeled as having "high-normal blood pressure."
Such a label, he feels, may segregate people unjustly into
a "near-hypertensive" category, a designation that might
eventually have negative implications for their job promo-
tions or for their insurance status. On the other hand, such
a designation might prove helpful if it serves to warn the
individual that he or she should make changes in diet,
exercise, or lifestyle.

Furthermore, the division of blood pressure classifications into mild and moderate levels may be subject to
some interpretation. Some physicians put those with 90 to
100 diastolic pressure into the "mild" classification. Their
"moderate" classification then becomes 101 to 114. Anything above that would be regarded as "severe." Doctors
who take this approach tend to be more aggressive in
prescribing nondrug strategies and medications earlier in
order to bring down the high blood pressure.

There are also some other ways to interpret the
meaning of blood pressure levels:

The Federal Aeronautics Administration is considerably more lenient than the Joint National Committee, at
least when it comes to determining who can fly commercial
airliners. To see what I mean, consider the following blood
pressure levels, which are regarded as acceptable for pilot
applicants when they are tested in a reclining position:

Age 20–29: 140/88

Age 30–39: 145/92

Age 40–49: 155/96

Age 50 and over: 160/98

Clearly, these standards allow those with established
high blood pressure to fly airliners. But why is such
hypertension allowed?

Probably the main reason is that the FAA places limits
on medications for pilots. So the choice has been made to
allow blood pressure to be a bit higher, rather than put a
cap on it with drugs.

Furthermore, another special dispensation may be
available to those applicants of at least 30 years of age

whose reclining blood pressure is higher than the maximum allowable for his or her age group. If the applicant undergoes a complete cardiovascular examination and is found to be normal, he or she can *still* qualify at the following blood pressure levels—which are even higher than those for regular applicants:

Age 30–39: 155/98

Age 40–49: 165/100

Age 50 and over: 170/100

When I first heard about these standards, I was shocked. In effect, these guidelines encourage the development of hypertension among one entire occupational group. These pilots may have to choose between their jobs and taking medications in amounts that will keep their hypertension at safe levels. Too often they choose the hypertension—and their employment as pilots.

So, we can see that the FAA has a radically different idea from the Joint National Committee about what is an acceptable level of blood pressure. In somewhat less dramatic fashion, there's also a significant difference of opinion between the American approach, reflected in the Joint National Committee's classifications and recommendations, and the practice of many British doctors.

In a 1987 British report, Dr. J. R. Hampton of the Department of Medicine, University Hospital, Queen's Medical Centre, Nottingham, argued that an "individual with a diastolic pressure of 100 mm Hg or less will certainly not gain any measurable benefit from drug therapy."

Furthermore, Dr. Hampton expressed skepticism about the justification for using medications to treat patients with diastolic pressures that go even higher. In particular, he said he believes "there is little evidence to support the treatment of patients with diastolic pressures up to 109 mm Hg. . . ."

Dr. Hampton acknowledges that treatment of diastolic pressures in the 100 to 109 range may reduce the risk of a stroke, but he says this benefit will "only be achieved at the price of side effects which may make the treatment unacceptable to a patient."

I happen to disagree with Dr. Hampton, as do the majority of American physicians, because I believe that the risks of serious cardiovascular events or organ damage far outweigh the possible side effects of medications.* In addition, there has been such progress in developing new drugs and in fine-tuning the application of older ones that side effects often can be minimized or eliminated.

But what Dr. Hampton's argument highlights is more important than any reservations I may have about his conclusions: In short, he—along with the FAA officials—points up the many possibilities of interpreting and treating blood pressure readings. This wide range of options can present some perplexing challenges for any physician, and can also be quite confusing for the patient who wants to understand and participate in his or her treatment.

Just how your doctor should go about measuring and evaluating your blood pressure—and how you can assist in this process—is our next concern.

How Is Your Blood Pressure Measured— And How Do You Know If It's Normal?

Whenever a patient has his blood pressure measured, I like to be sure that he understands these basic principles at the outset:

Principle 1. Don't assume that you know what your blood pressure really is after one reading or even one set of readings.

---

* The 1970 VA Cooperative Study showed that there was a definite advantage in treating moderate hypertension (diastolic blood pressure of 105 to 114 mm Hg), the advantage being primarily in the prevention of stroke and congestive heart failure rather than coronary artery disease.

True blood pressure has to be ascertained over a period of time and in a variety of circumstances. Also, to catch any changes in pressure, regular checks over the years are essential.

What are the practical implications of this principle? Simply this: Your pressure should be checked every time you have a complete physical exam, or *at least once every two years* if your doctor finds in one exam that you're in the normal range.

On the other hand, if your physician determines that your diastolic (lower) reading is in the high-normal range (85 to 89 according to the Joint National Committee's classifications), you should be rechecked within one year.

If your diastolic reading is in the 90 to 104 category, or if your systolic is in the 140 to 199 range, you should come back for another evaluation within two months. If your diastolic is measured at 105 to 114, or if your systolic is 200 or higher, your physician should evaluate you further or refer you to special care within two weeks. Finally, if your diastolic is 115 or above, your doctor should evaluate you further or refer you immediately to special care.

Principle 2. Don't panic if you have one high reading.

There are many reasons for one high reading, or one set of high readings—including the white-coat syndrome, which we will discuss in more detail shortly. It's true that a person with one high reading is, statistically, more at risk for having or developing hypertension; at the same time, however, *many* people have one high reading in the doctor's office but then find, through further testing, that they don't have a problem.

In addition, high blood pressure is only *one* risk factor for various cardiovascular problems. Hypertension alone is certainly a concern, but not as much a concern if it's all that's wrong with you. So, if your cholesterol is high or out of balance, and if you're overweight, if you smoke, or if you lead a sedentary lifestyle—then high blood pressure puts you at higher risk than if you didn't have these other risk factors.

If your blood pressure measurement is high, your physician will likely begin a series of further checks and rechecks to determine the accuracy of the first reading. In the meantime, just relax and wait for the final evaluation to come in.

Remember: *Everyone*'s blood pressure fluctuates to some extent on an hour-by-hour and minute-by-minute basis, depending on the intensity of activity and stress levels. Furthermore, many people experience relatively dramatic rises and drops in blood pressure during the course of a day—but again, that doesn't necessarily mean that these people are hypertensive.

Principle 3. Your average blood pressure is the key to an accurate evaluation.

Your physician should always take at least two to three readings during your physical exam, and then find the average.

The Joint National Committee recommends finding the average of only two readings. But they say that if those two vary by more than 5 mm Hg, additional measurements should be taken.

My special consultant, Dr. Norman Kaplan, recommends a set of three readings for each exam, and I concur with this approach for two reasons: First, taking one extra reading for all exams appears to enhance the accuracy of the final average measurement; second, it is much easier for doctors to make a standard practice of taking three readings, without qualification, rather than to say that in some cases two should be taken and in other cases more may be required.

Now, assume that your doctor finds that your first average blood pressure measurement is sufficiently high to have you come in for a recheck within two months. In such a case, he should take a total of at least three groups of readings during those two months, with two weeks or more between each group. Once again, he'll average all these readings to get a more accurate picture of your blood pressure.

(*Note:* Your doctor may want you to participate in finding your blood pressure average by taking home readings on a home monitoring device. We'll discuss these home gadgets later in this chapter.)

• • •

Principle 4. Your risk from high blood pressure is on a continuum.

One of the reasons it's so hard to classify a person according to a blood pressure range or category is that the risks from hypertension—including stroke, kidney failure, and other organ damage—increase gradually, as the average blood pressure level rises.

In other words, a person with a 140/90 reading may have hypertension according to the latest definitions, but he's at a lower level of risk than a person with 150/95; and a person with a measurement of 160/100 is at an even higher risk.

An important corollary of this principle is that you should count it a success when your doctor is able to bring your blood pressure down even a little bit!

A second corollary is that you shouldn't despair or panic if your doctor cannot bring your blood pressure down to normal levels immediately through medications or nondrug means. Because the damage caused by hypertension occurs so slowly, you probably have time for your physician to try a variety of treatments until he finds the right one for you.

A third corollary is that, in general, blood pressure cannot be too low. But there are some exceptions:

- The patient may be in shock, as may occur after a serious accident.

- The patient may have *hypo*tension (blood pressure so low that he or she begins to experience weakness, dizziness, or other problems).

- The patient may be in an advanced state of alcoholism, with the condition known as Wernicke's syndrome. In this case, systolic blood pressure commonly drops to 50 to 60 mm Hg, with no signs of hypotension.

But aside from these special problems, there's nothing wrong with very low blood pressure. In this regard, I'm reminded of one perfectly healthy woman whose typical average blood pressure readings are about 85/60. No, that's not a misprint! Her readings *are* that low—a systolic of 85 and a diastolic of 60. Some people might have the symptoms of hypotension at these levels, but not this woman. She's completely symptom-free, and she's at a much lower risk for hypertension and its related problems than are those whose blood pressure is 140/90 or above.

With these principles firmly in mind, let's assume that you're ready to go to your doctor's office for a blood pressure reading. Following are the basic guidelines:

- You should avoid smoking, consuming caffeine, or eating before the test.

- Avoid anxiety-producing activities or thoughts. If you're sensitive to stress, these anxieties will show up on the measurement.

- Don't do anything that involves heavy exertion—especially isometric (muscle-tensing) exercises—immediately before the test.

- Avoid becoming chilled or overly cold just prior to the exam. This will cause your muscles to tense and may increase blood pressure levels.

- Urinate before you go into the doctor's examining room. A full bladder may raise your readings.

- Tell your doctor if you are on any medications, including adrenal steroids, estrogens, or over-the-counter drugs such as nose drops. These may elevate blood pressure levels.

- You should be seated, leaning back with your spine relaxed and comfortable against the chair. Your arm should be bared and supported at heart level, either by the chair arm or by some other flat surface. Studies have shown that an arm hanging down at the side, rather than being supported at heart level, can raise pressures by 10 to 12 points.

    Another common mistake that's made in many examining rooms—and that may raise your blood pressure levels significantly—is to allow the patient in effect to do isometric exercises as his blood pressure is being taken. There are several ways this can happen:

First, if the back isn't supported, tension develops in the back muscles. One study revealed that readings were as much as 10 points higher for patients without back supports.

Second, if the arm isn't supported, the muscles in the arm may tense and contribute to a rise in pressure—by as much as 10 percent, according to one report.

Third, any other muscle that is tense will cause a rise in pressure. So, both the physician and the patient should check to be sure that every part of the patient's body is completely relaxed and supported by means other than muscle power.

- Avoid talking while the test is being conducted, as conversation may raise your blood pressure above levels that occur when you're quiet.

- You should rest quietly in the examining chair for at least five minutes before your pressure is taken.

- The cuff of the blood pressure device (the mercury sphygmomanometer) should fit properly. Specifically, the rubber bladder of the device should encircle at least two-thirds of your arm. If the cuff size isn't right—i.e., if the patient's arm is too small, as with a child, or too large, as with a large adult—other sizes should be made available.

- On a first visit, the doctor may measure your pressure while you're standing and also lying on your back (supine). This technique is most common when the patient is elderly or diabetic.

- On an initial visit, the doctor will usually check the pressure in both of your arms, and if there's a difference, he'll choose the arm with the higher pressure. To determine whether both arms are the same, the physician may simply do a quick check of the pulse in each arm; if they are the same, he'll do a formal test on only one arm.

- The doctor must measure both your systolic (upper) blood pressure and your diastolic (lower) pressure.

He finds these readings by pumping up the inflatable bladder on the cuff device rapidly until your pulse at the wrist disappears. Then, after the pulse disappears, the physician will listen through his stethoscope as he begins to deflate the bladder slowly, at a rate of 2 to 3 mm Hg per heartbeat (or per second).

When he reaches a certain point in this deflation process, the blood will begin to rush back into the closed-off vessels. This flow will cause a kind of tapping or thumping sound in the stethoscope—a sound known as "Korotkoff phase I," named for the well-known hypertension researcher in the early twentieth century.

This first sound signals the point at which the body's blood pressure overcomes the resistance from the cuff on the arm. Most important for purposes of measurement, it's the marker for the systolic blood pressure reading. The physician can tell what number should be assigned to the onset of this sound by checking the mercury level or dial on the sphygmomanometer. So, if the tapping sound begins when the gauge registers "130," then the systolic blood pressure of the patient is recorded as 130 mm Hg (millimeters of mercury).

But this is only the first part of the measurement process. The physician continues to listen to the tapping sounds through his stethoscope until they stop. Precisely at the point that they cease—known as "Korotkoff phase V"—the physician notes the reading on the mercury level or dial. This figure represents the diastolic blood pressure, or the pressure on the vessels when the heart is at rest, filling up with blood and preparing for the next pumping action.

So, in our hypothetical case, the patient's diastolic number might be 80. His complete reading, then, would be a quite normal 130/80, read as "one thirty over eighty."

In most cases this procedure produces valid results, at least for one set of readings. But there are exceptions, one of which is the condition known as "pseudohypertension."

Pseudohypertension occasionally occurs among people who have rigid or calcified vessels, and especially among older patients. With these people, the inflated cuff-and-bladder device may not be able to collapse the rigid artery until the pressure in the bladder is well above the true systolic pressure inside the artery. The reading on the sphygmomanometer may then be considerably higher than the patient's true blood pressure. The doctor usually recognizes this condition when he continues to feel a pulse in the rigid artery even after the cuff has collapsed the artery farther up in the arm.

One 65-year-old woman had a blood pressure reading of 240/120—a dangerously high level normally requiring immediate medical intervention. But on further examination her physician noticed that there was still a pulse in her arm; the blood vessels were apparently so rigid (calcified) that they remained open even when no blood was flowing into them.

The physician wanted to be certain that her very high readings were not related simply to her rigid vessels. So he took an intra-arterial blood pressure reading by inserting a needle into the woman's arm. This time, the true blood pressure, 180/85, came to light. The systolic pressure was still too high, but it wasn't at a dangerous level; and the diastolic reading was normal.

Another situation that can cause confusion about blood pressure readings is a measurement that is very low—even zero in a few cases!—on the diastolic (lower) reading. Those suffering from anemia or from vitamin B-1 deficiency—and also some otherwise healthy pregnant women, young children, and people who have a great deal of anxiety—may have clear systolic readings, which can be detected easily through the blood pressure device. But the tapping sound of the blood rushing back into the arm may continue far beyond what's considered normal, so that the diastolic pressure comes in at 50 or even lower. (Remember: A doctor determines diastolic blood pressure by listening for the point when the tapping sound in his stethoscope *stops.*)

Sometimes the continuation of the tapping sound may be due to mechanical or technical problems. For example, the physician may be holding the stethoscope on the cuff device too hard over the artery in the upper arm. All the doctor has to do is release the pressure he's applying to the stethoscope, and the tapping will end, thus giving him the diastolic reading.

At other times, a muffled sound may occur and never disappear. In this situation, the physician should note the time when the clear tapping ends and the muffled sounds begin, and take that point to be the diastolic pressure.

On the other hand, there are situations in which these procedural adjustments don't change anything, and the tapping sounds never stop. Consequently, the diastolic pressure appears to be at or near zero—even though the patient seems quite healthy.

Sometimes these very low blood pressure readings are normal for the particular individual—though obviously they are highly unusual when compared with pressures of most people. It is up to the physician to determine whether a patient fits into this unusual-but-healthy category.

Many times, however, other measuring devices may reveal a diastolic pressure that for some reason wasn't picked up by the sphygmomanometer. In one such case, a woman in her fifties had a systolic pressure of 175, but a diastolic pressure of zero. No matter what adjustments the physician made in his equipment and technique, he still ended up with that zero reading.

Finally, he asked her to use a home monitoring device with a digital readout of pressure levels. Probably because the home device detected the movement of blood within the artery under the cuff rather than picking up the korotkoff sounds, the measurement came out as 175/90.

This revealed a hypertensive condition, but one that could be dealt with initially through nondrug treatments. An intra-artery test of her blood pressure later confirmed this reading.

Such home monitoring devices have proved useful time and time again as physicians try to determine the true blood pressure levels of their patients. Used wisely, these gadgets are prime examples of how cooperation between patient and physician can enhance the evaluation and treatment of hypertension.

3

Control Through Exercise

Regular aerobic exercise—such as jogging, running, cycling, and swimming—is one of the most effective nondrug "medicines" for those at risk for hypertension.

But exactly what kind of aerobics program should you try—and, just as important, what kinds of exercise should you avoid?

Although an intelligently designed aerobics program will often help lower blood pressure, some types of physical activity may work *against* your attempt to control your hypertension.

For example, infrequent workouts usually have no beneficial impact on blood pressure. In addition, some muscle-tensing activities, such as weight lifting, may be even dangerous for those with hypertension.

Further, certain people with severe hypertension shouldn't do *any* strenuous exercise unless their blood pressure can be controlled with drugs. This is because athletic activity may trigger a serious health complication, like a stroke, for those whose blood pressure remains too high.

I've established a limit of 175/110 mm Hg for my patients. In other words, if a person's systolic or diastolic measurement doesn't drop below that level with medications, I don't permit vigorous exercise. Even at lower levels of hypertension, the decision regarding exercise should be made by a physician.

Another complexity in this picture is the question of exercise while taking beta-blocker medications. These drugs reduce the blood pressure by lowering the heart rate. But working out with a significantly lowered heart rate will affect performance, cause symptoms in some people, and definitely place a limit on the aerobic effect achievable by beta-blocker-treated patients.

To get the maximum benefit from exercise under such conditions, it's helpful to make use of a special formula for determining the target heart rate, which I'll discuss later.

Now, let's examine more closely what happens to blood pressure during different types of exercise.

What Happens to Blood Pressure During Aerobic Exercise

Either the systolic or the diastolic blood pressure, or both, go up during exercise. But the short-term *and* long-term responses of blood pressure can vary considerably, depending on the type of exercise in which the person engages and upon his or her overall health and physical fitness.

For example, a highly conditioned 21-year-old who was examined at the Aerobics Center was found to have a normal blood pressure of 114/72 mm Hg before he exercised on the treadmill.

As he began to walk and the work load increased, his systolic pressure rose steadily. During this first phase of the exercise, which lasted about twenty-five minutes, he was exercising aerobically. That is, he was consuming oxygen at about the same rate as he was expending it.

But by the thirtieth minute, he was exercising *an*aerobically—he was expending more oxygen than he was able to take in. At this point, he attained a maximum heart rate of 195 beats per minute, and a systolic blood pressure of 220 mm Hg. Finally, he was unable to continue because of exhaustion.

His diastolic pressure during the test dropped to a level lower than at the baseline (his initial, resting blood pressure measurement)—or about 60 mm Hg. This rise in the systolic but decline in the diastolic pressure during exercise is typical of a well-conditioned athlete of any age.

Also, note that both the systolic and diastolic pressures continued to decline during the ten-minute recovery. In fact, in the post-exercise resting phase, it's not uncommon for both the systolic and diastolic pressures to drop below their baseline levels in highly conditioned subjects.

Other clinical observations have revealed that these lower levels of blood pressure after exercise may persist for a half hour or longer. Then, the measurements creep back up to the original, baseline levels.

Normal Blood Pressure Response in a Highly Conditioned Man

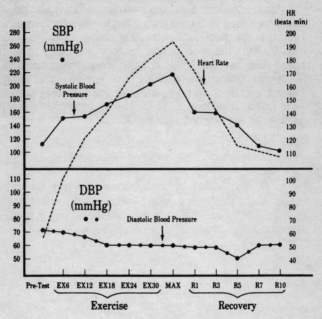

Treadmill Time (Min)

In my second example, the patient is a true "vascular reactor." In particular, he suffers from the "white-coat" or "doctor's office" syndrome. This man is highly conditioned, as indicated by his treadmill performance, which exceeded twenty-five minutes. But *prior* to stress testing, his systolic blood pressure was elevated at 170/74, and his heart rate was 80. In such a fit person, I would have expected a heart rate lower than 60, and also a lower systolic pressure.

As he began to exercise, the systolic increased only minimally. In fact, at ten minutes on the treadmill, the systolic reading was identical to what it had been at rest, despite the substantial increase in heart rate.

At maximal performance, his blood pressure peaked at 240/60. Then, ten minutes into recovery, the measurement dropped to 139/68, a level slightly higher than his average daily pressure, which had been ascertained during a twenty-four-hour monitoring program. Aerobic exercise, in other words, had lowered his sensitive blood pressure back to normal.

In light of cases like this, I often suggest to my true "vascular reactors" that they exercise *before* having a blood pressure measurement. Such preliminary exercise and the physical fatigue that accompanies it typically eliminate any "emotional" response associated with the white-coat phenomenon.

Another related point: In those with true hypertension, a post-exercise normal blood pressure, though temporary, *may* signal that exercise will be effective in treating hypertension—and that drugs may not be required.

A "Vascular Reactor" with "White-Coat" Syndrome (Systolic Pressure Only)

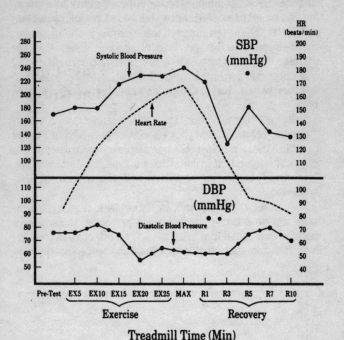

Treadmill Time (Min)

My next illustration involves another type of "vascular reactivity," but one limited to changes in the *diastolic* pressure. When this person was at rest immediately prior to stress testing, his pressure was elevated at 140/100. But the patient was in outstanding physical condition, as indicated by the time he was able to stay on the treadmill (more than twenty-five minutes).

At peak exercise, his blood pressure was 210/65, and

the diastolic pressure had steadily decreased. Ten minutes into recovery, his blood pressure was 118/70.

In this case, as in the preceding one, exercising moderately *before* having the blood pressure determined might have normalized the patient's pressure (in this instance, the diastolic pressure). Again, twenty-four-hour monitoring revealed that there was no persistent elevation during the day.

A "Vascular Reactor" with "White-Coat" Syndrome (Diastolic Elevation Only)

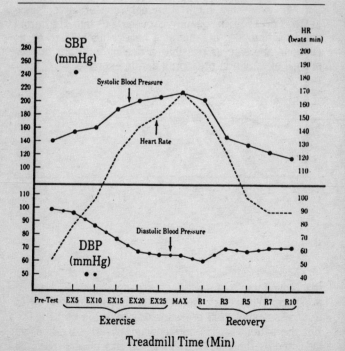

Treadmill Time (Min)

In true hypertension, as reflected in the next graph, the blood pressure is elevated at rest (i.e., 140/102 mm Hg). With exercise in this case, the systolic pressure increases substantially, to levels of 260 mm Hg or higher. Then, during recovery, it drops only to the preexercise level.

The diastolic pressure in this third example doesn't change substantially.

Note: The maximum blood pressure usually considered acceptable during exercise is 240/120 mm Hg. Unless the physician is familiar with the patient (as was the situation here), I recommend termination of an exercise test or of a workout if either the systolic or diastolic levels exceed those values.

My view may seem extremely conservative, since systolic pressure frequently exceeds 240 mm Hg during weight lifting. But in general, I believe it's best to be as cautious and safe as possible in dealing with any above-normal elevation in pressures during exercise.

The Blood Pressure Response to Exercise in a Patient with True Hypertension

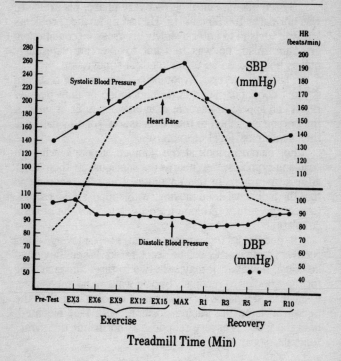

Treadmill Time (Min)

Among people who are in poor physical condition, the blood pressure response following maximal performance may involve symptoms of hypotension or near-fainting. In the following graph, you can see that the preexercise blood pressure in one such case was low normal, at 90/70 mm Hg. In response to exercise, the systolic pressure steadily increased, but peaked at only 158 mm Hg, whereas the diastolic pressure steadily declined.

During recovery, the systolic pressure dropped immediately to below 80 mm Hg. As a result, the walking cool-down had to be stopped to prevent the patient from fainting. He was then placed in the supine position, at which point his pressure began to rise.

By ten minutes into the recovery phase, his pressure was normal at 100/50 mm Hg. He had no further problems but was advised to enter a slowly progressive conditioning program. Also, he was told not to exercise vigorously unless he could do so under medical supervision.

This post-exercise, hypotensive, near-fainting response is most commonly seen in deconditioned or unfit people. But it can appear in anyone, man or woman, fit or unfit, if the person is pushed to total exhaustion—or to what I call the "supermax" level of exercise.

For instance, look at the number of people who are "walking zombies," or nearly unconscious on their feet, after a marathon. In this condition, I usually recommend that the individual keep moving, with support if necessary, to help the return of blood from the legs into the general circulation.

If people in this situation can keep moving, their recovery time usually will be accelerated. When they must lie down, however, it may take two to three times as long for their bodies to readjust. Should walking be impossible, even in a stooped-over position, I recommend that the person assume the supine position, with feet elevated, until the blood pressure response is normal or the symptoms disappear.

The Hypotensive or Near-Fainting Response with Exercise

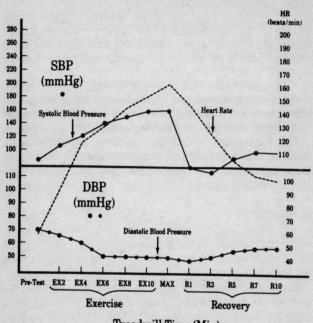

Treadmill Time (Min)

A rare but potentially dangerous blood pressure response sometimes occurs while taking a stress test. Called "cardiac or heart decompensation with exercise," this condition is characterized by decreasing heart rate and systolic blood pressure, even in the presence of an increasing work load. (See the following graph.)

Notice that the patient whose case is presented there walked twelve minutes on the treadmill, but that he reached the peak systolic pressure at five minutes and peak heart rate at eight minutes.

Unless the physician is very familiar with the patient, I advise that the stress test be discontinued whenever the heart rate or systolic pressure begins to drop with demanding exercise. If the exercise isn't stopped, cardiac failure can occur abruptly.

The physical condition of this patient, which *was* well known to the physician, didn't lead to any problems during this particular test or later. You'll also notice that the blood pressure and heart rate responses during recovery were normal.

In teaching physicians proper treadmill stress-testing techniques, I always use this patient's response as an example of an "abnormal" test, even though the electrocardiogram may be completely normal. The majority of such patients have underlying, moderate to severe heart disease, and their exercise programs must be limited to participation in cardiac rehabilitation classes.

Cardiac Decompensation Occurring with Exercise

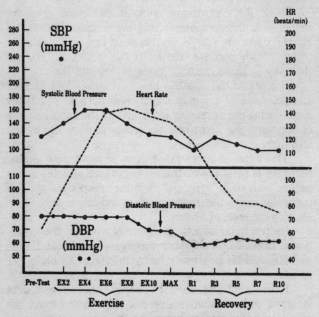

Treadmill Time (Min)

In my final examples, I want to document the heart rate and blood pressure responses in two men, 50 years of age, one in average physical condition, the other a highly competitive masters runner.

In the first example—the man in average shape—the blood pressure at rest is normal (120/80 mm Hg), and the heart rate is 68 beats per minute. Both the heart rate and blood pressure in this patient increase steadily with exercise, reaching a maximum of 180 beats per minute and a systolic reading of 190 mm Hg. The diastolic pressure remains relatively stable.

During recovery, however, the heart rate drops slowly, and at the five-minute mark it's still 110 (the heart rate should be under 100 for people over 50 years of age). At ten minutes into recovery, the heart rate continues to be slightly elevated at 100, but the blood pressure is normal at 120/70.

Now, for comparison, look at the blood pressure response in the competitive masters runner. At rest, his blood pressure is 122/78, and his heart rate is 50 beats per minute. With exercise, the heart rate peaks at 170, and the systolic blood pressure rises to 200 mm Hg.

But notice the diastolic blood pressure: In a manner characteristic of a highly conditioned person, it actually *drops* during the increasing work load. In the initial minutes of recovery, the heart rate decreases rapidly, and by the fifth minute it's only 85.

This type of accelerated drop in heart rate during recovery is seen in well-trained endurance athletes and in people with near-"syncopal" (fainting) responses. In this particular case, the readings were indicative only of an exceptional level of fitness.

By ten minutes into the recovery phase, the conditioned man's blood pressure was again normal, at 120/68 mm Hg, and his heart rate had stabilized at 85 beats per minute.

Because of the need to "repay" the oxygen debt incurred with exhaustive exercise, you can't expect the recovery heart rate to return to the preexercise levels until one and a half or two hours have elapsed. (But note: There's a continuing benefit with the higher heart rate. Your body continues to burn calories during the recovery that follows exhaustive and demanding exercise!)

Blood Pressure and Heart Rate Response (A 50-Year-Old Man in Average Condition)

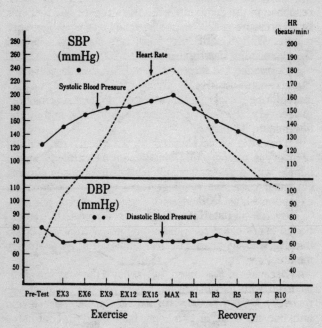

Treadmill Time (Min)

Blood Pressure and Heart Rate Response (A Highly Conditioned 50-Year-Old Man)

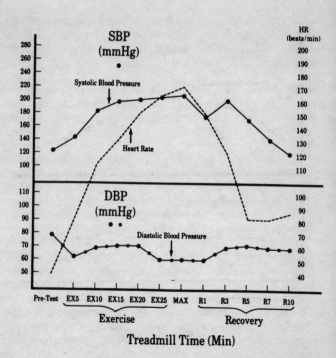

The dangers of isometric exercise. Any exercise that involves relatively static tensing of the muscles over a period of several seconds is known as isometric exercise. The most common examples of this type of activity include weight training, or the lifting of any heavy object. In fact, calisthenics, such as push-ups or supine straight leg lifts, may have an isometric component and should be avoided by those with uncontrolled hypertension.

There are recorded instances of the blood pressure of weight lifters increasing to levels as high as 300/150 or even higher during a maximum lift. Obviously, such an upward surge of pressure is potentially dangerous for anyone with hypertension. And even for healthy, nonhypertensive people, intense isometric exercise may present a problem.

Take the case of a 17-year-old athlete who went in for a routine, preseason checkup. He was in great physical shape, with a low percentage of body fat and a high level of aerobic, or cardiovascular, fitness.

On the other hand, his blood pressure at rest was 150/85 mm Hg. This diastolic measurement was in the upper range of normal, and the systolic pressure was also slightly elevated. (The suggested upper limits of blood pressure for children 14 to 18 years of age are 135/90 mm Hg.)

This young patient's systolic pressure—according to the 1988 Joint National Committee's guidelines for hypertension among young people—placed him in the 99th percentile for systolic pressure among all 16-to-18-year-olds. Such a measurement qualified this adolescent as potentially at risk for significant systolic hypertension.

Later exams during the next one to two months confirmed that the boy did indeed have a high systolic blood pressure. In addition, the readings were not the result of the "white-coat" phenomenon: during the preceding two annual exams, his pressure had been normal.

Upon further questioning, the doctor learned that the boy had engaged in heavy weight training during the past two years, and even more vigorously throughout the preceding summer.

The physician determined that this weight training was the *only* unusual risk factor that might account for his hypertension. Consequently, he requested that the boy discontinue his weight training entirely and concentrate on aerobic activities such as running.

This recommendation met with some resistance because the youngster wanted to be as big and strong as possible for football. But he finally complied with his doctor's advice.

When the boy's blood pressure was reevaluated a month later, both the systolic and diastolic readings had begun to decline. They continued to drop even more during the succeeding months as the boy minimized his weight training.

Note: This example *doesn't* mean that all weight training causes hypertension. But frequent blood pressure monitoring should be done for those who engage in heavy weight lifting.

The higher blood pressure produced by isometric exercise has been confirmed in a number of studies, including one reported in the *Archives of Internal Medicine* in 1984. There, researcher M. H. Maxwell and several other investigators compared the differences in blood pressure responses among normotensive patients who engaged first in aerobic exercise, then in isometric exercise.

The scientists discovered that when the participants did isometric exercises, systolic pressure increased from an average of 120 to more than 220 mm Hg. The diastolic pressure increased from slightly above 80 to an average of 140 mm Hg.

In contrast, when the participants engaged in aerobic activity, the systolic pressure increased from 120 to 180 mm Hg. The difference in diastolic readings was even more dramatic: the diastolic pressures of the aerobic exercisers actually *declined* from an average of 80 to well below 60 mm Hg! (You'll note that this finding is consistent with our report from the Aerobics Center, illustrated on page 34 earlier in this chapter.)

My conclusion: Since there is an exaggerated increase in both the systolic and diastolic blood pressures during heavy weight lifting, such activity should be avoided both by hypertensives *and* by those with normal blood pressure.

On the other hand, aerobic (endurance-type) exercise

has been shown to have the opposite effect, as we'll see in the following section.

Endurance Exercise Can Lower Blood Pressure

Many studies have demonstrated the benefits of aerobic exercise in lowering blood pressure.

Recognizing these findings, an article published in "Hypertension," the 1988 Consensus Conference on Exercise, Fitness and Health reported: "Individuals with essential hypertension can decrease their resting systolic and diastolic blood pressure by approximately 10 mm Hg with endurance exercise training."

Here's an example of how this principle can work:

A 40-year-old man weighed 169 pounds and had a blood pressure reading of 118/91 mm Hg—i.e., a mildly elevated diastolic pressure. Subsequently, he embarked on an exercise program designed by Dr. Salah el-Dean and colleagues at the School of Pharmacy at the University of Mississippi. The program required the participant to begin exercising on a rowing machine for fifteen minutes three times a week, with a gradual increase in rowing time to forty-five minutes per session.

After seven months, this man experienced an 8 percent decline in weight. Also, his blood pressure dropped to 111/81, or well within the normal range.

Although this is a single case history, similar results have been reported frequently, both in ordinary clinical situations and in larger studies. For example:

- The 1988 U.S. Railroad Study found that over a twenty-year period, middle-aged men with lower levels of physical fitness—as revealed by their higher heart rates during submaximal exercise—are at greater risk of dying from coronary heart disease, cardiovascular disease, and other causes. Most important for our purposes, these researchers noted that the higher death risk for these men is *"largely due to higher blood pressure levels."* (Emphasis by Dr. Cooper.)

- During a sixteen-week aerobic exercise program conducted at the Aerobics Center in Dallas, endurance exercise significantly lowered the blood pressure of mildly hypertensive patients.

  Investigator John Duncan and several colleagues, reporting in the *Journal of the American Medical Association,* found that the systolic pressures dropped from an average of 146.3 to 133.9 mm Hg, and the diastolic readings from 94.3 to 87.2 mm Hg.

  The exercise program utilized in this study consisted of three one-hour sessions per week and included the following activities: (1) a 10 to 15 minute warm-up; (2) a walking and jogging phase of about 40 minutes, at 70 to 80 percent of maximal heart rate; and (3) a 10-minute cool-down period. As the program progressed and the participants achieved higher levels of fitness, the jogging was increased and the walking was decreased.

- Twelve hypertensive Japanese patients were placed on a mild aerobic exercise program for ten to twenty weeks, according to researcher Akira Kiyonaga's report in the journal *Hypertension.*

  The results: There was a significant reduction in plasma catecholamine levels. Also, after ten weeks, the researchers noted a reduction in average systolic/diastolic pressures of more than 20/10 mm Hg in 50 percent of the patients. After the full twenty-week program, 78 percent of the participants experienced a similar reduction in blood pressure.

Clearly, then, the cardiovascular fitness produced by aerobic exercise can have a beneficial effect on lowering blood pressure. However, patients on antihypertensive medications such as beta blockers, which limit heart rate, have sometimes found it difficult to achieve higher levels of cardiovascular fitness. What can be done for them?

Exercise Programs as Therapy for Hypertension

The following exercises are recommended especially for those who have been diagnosed with hypertension or who have a tendency to develop it.

I've purposely excluded exercises that require tensing or straining, such as heavy weight training or highly resistant calisthenics (such as push-ups). These are known to raise blood pressure levels. Yet, if your hypertension is only mild, your physician may allow or even recommend light muscle-building activities.

For example, you may be at risk for osteoporosis. Therefore, your doctor may feel that even though you are mildly hypertensive, you should engage in additional weight-bearing exercises to increase your bone density. I've included a number of such exercises in my book *Preventing Osteoporosis*.

However, any decision to add weight-bearing exercises to the suggested programs should be made *only* in consultation with your physician.

Following are four other guidelines you should follow with these exercise programs:

1. Remember—blood pressure measurements greater than 175/110 mm Hg, with or without medication, are a *contraindication* to *any* vigorous exercise program. Only when *both* the systolic and diastolic readings can be controlled with medication is vigorous exercise permitted. **Important:** This limitation includes the exercise programs found in this book as well as those from other sources.

2. Be sure to have a thorough physical exam before embarking on this program. If hypertension is diagnosed, proceed only with the full knowledge and supervision of your physician.

3. If your blood pressure is 160/105 or higher, begin an exercise program *only* after your doctor has started you on appropriate drug therapy. Your response to such therapy will determine the point at which you can embark on an exercise program.

4. If you are on drugs for hypertension when you begin this program, reduce the dosages of those drugs *only* with the permission of your physician.

The Exercise Program for Hypertension

Walking

| | | Time Goals (min) | | | | |
| | | Age (years) | | | | |
Week	Distance (miles)	<30	30–49	50–59	60+	Freq/wk
1	1.0	16:00	17:00	19:00	22:00	4–5x
2	1.0	14:00	15:00	17:00	20:00	4–5x
3	1.5	22:00	24:00	26:00	30:00	4–5x
4	1.5	21:00	23:00	25:00	29:00	4–5x
5	2.0	29:00	32:00	34:00	39:00	4–5x
6	2.0	28:00	31:00	33:00	38:00	4–5x
7	2.5	36:00	40:00	42:00	48:00	4–5x
8	2.5	35:00	39:00	41:00	47:00	4–5x
9	3.0	43:00	48:00	50:00	57:00	4–5x
10	3.0	42:30	47:00	49:00	55:00	4–5x
11	3.0	42:00	46:00	48:00	53:00	4–5x
12	3.0	<42:00	<45:00	<47:00	<51:00	3–4x

By week 12, an adequate aerobic fitness level has been reached and should be maintained by walking the prescribed distance in the allotted time. Exercising four to five times per week is recommended, but even three times per week is enough to assure a satisfactory level of fitness.

<Means "less than."

Swimming

		Time Goals (min)				
	Distance	Age (years)				
Week	(yards)	<30	30–49	50–59	60+	Freq/wk
1	200	6:00	7:00	8:00	8:00	4–5x
2	300	9:00	9:30	10:00	11:00	4–5x
3	400	12:00	12:00	13:00	14:00	4–5x
4	450	13:00	13:00	14:00	15:00	4–5x
5	500	14:00	14:00	15:00	16:00	4–5x
6	600	16:00	17:00	18:00	19:00	4–5x
7	600	skip	skip	17:00	18:00	4–5x
8	700	18:00	19:00	20:00	21:00	4–5x
9	700	skip	skip	19:30	20:00	4–5x
10	800	20:00	21:00	22:00	23:00	3–4x
11	900	22:30	24:00	25:00	26:00	3–4x
12	1000	<25:00	<26:30	<28:00	<30:00	3–4x

Use the stroke that enables you to swim the required distance in the allotted time. During the initial weeks, rest when necessary (this is taken into consideration in the time goals). The programs for the under 30 and 30 to 39 age groups are only 10 weeks in duration, so skip the weeks indicated. Try to reach the time goals by the end of the week and if the goal cannot be reached, repeat the week.

The three stretching exercises used in conjunction with the Aqua-Aerobics Program (see p. 58) should be used prior to beginning to swim.

<Means "less than."

Stationary Cycling

		Time Goals (min)				
	Speed	Age (years)				
Week	(mph/rpm)	<30	30–49	50–59	60 +	Freq/wk
1	15/55	8:00	6:00	5:00	4:00	4–5x
2	15/55	10:00	8:00	7:00	6:00	4–5x
3	15/55	12:00	10:00	9:00	8:00	4–5x
4	17.5/65	14:00	12:00	11:00	10:00	4–5x
5	17.5/65	16:00	14:00	13:00	12:00	4–5x
6	17.5/65	18:00	16:00	15:00	14:00	4–5x
7	17.5/65	20:00	18:00	17:00	16:00	4–5x
8	17.5/65	22:00	20:00	19:00	18:00	4–5x
9	20/75	24:00	22:00	21:00	20:00	4–5x
10	20/75	26:00	24:00	23:00	22:00	4–5x
11	25/90	28:00	26:00	25:00	24:00	4–5x
12	25/90	30:00	28:00	27:00	25:00	4–5x

During the first 6 weeks, warm up by cycling slowly for 3 minutes, at 18 to 20 mph, with no resistance, before beginning the actual workout. At the conclusion of the exercise, cool down by cycling for 3 minutes without resistance.

Add enough resistance or cycle fast enough that the pulse rate counted for 10 seconds immediately after exercise and multiplied by 6 equals these heart rates:

Patients Not on Beta Blockers

Less than 30 years of age	140–160
30–49 years of age	135–155
50–59 years of age	130–150
60 + years of age	110–130

Patients on Beta Blockers

Those on beta blockers should adjust their heart rates accordingly. If the pulse rate is higher, lower the resistance before exercising again; if it is lower, increase the resistance.

Treadmill Walking

| | | | Time Goals (min) | | | | |
| | | | Age (years) | | | | |
Week	Speed (mph)	Incline (%)	<30	30–49	50–59	60 +	Freq/wk
1	3.0	0%	20:00	18:00	15:00	10:00	4–5x
2	3.0	0%	20:00	18:00	16:00	12:00	4–5x
3	3.25	0%	20:00	18:00	16:00	12:00	4–5x
4	3.25	0%	22:00	20:00	18:00	14:00	4–5x
5	3.5	0%	22:00	20:00	18:00	15:00	4–5x
6	3.5	5%	24:00	22:00*	20:00*	16:00*	4–5x
7	4.0	5%	24:00	22:00	20:00	16:00	4–5x
8	4.0	7½%	26:00	24:00	22:00	18:00	4–5x
9	4.0	7½%	28:00	26:00	24:00	20:00	4–5x
10	4.0	10%	30:00	28:00	25:00	22:00	4–5x

*Beginning with week 6, the following inclines can be used to increase the work load and aerobic benefit:

Age (years)

Week	30–49	50–59	60 +
6	5%	2½%	0%
7	5%	2½%	0%
8	7½%	5%	2½%
9	7½%	5%	2½%
10	10%	7½%	5%

Always warm up for 3 to 5 minutes at 2 mph, no incline, and cool down for 5 minutes at 2 mph, no incline.

These programs assume that the treadmill is motor driven, not self-propelled.

Exercising four to five times per week is recommended, but even three times per week is enough to assure a satisfactory level of fitness.

Cycling (outdoors)

Week	Distance (miles)	Time Goals (min) Age (years) <30	30–49	50–59	60 + *	Freq/wk
1	4.0	24:00	25:00	27:00	30:00	4–5x
2	4.0	22:00	23:00	25:00	28:00	4–5x
3	4.0	20:00	22:00	24:00	27:00	4–5x
4	5.0	28:00	30:00	32:00	36:00	4–5x
5	5.0	26:00	29:00	31:00	35:00	4–5x
6	5.0	24:00	27:00	29:00	34:00	4–5x
7	6.0	32:00	36:00	38:00	44:00	4–5x
8	6.0	30:00	34:00	36:00	42:00	4–5x
9	6.0	28:00	33:00	35:00	40:00	4–5x
10	7.0	37:00	41:00	44:00	49:00	4–5x
11	7.0	35:00	38:00	41:00	47:00	4–5x
12	7.0	<33:00	<35:00	<38:00	<45:00	4–5x

By week 12, an adequate level of aerobic fitness has been reached and should be maintained by cycling the prescribed distance in the allotted time. Exercising four to five times per week is recommended. But even three times per week is enough to assure a satisfactory level of fitness.

*Cycling outdoors is not usually recommended for the totally inactive person past 60 years of age. But when a regular cyclist reaches 60, it is recommended that the cycling be continued without restrictions. To avoid problems including falls and fractures, three-wheeled cycling is encouraged, and this progressive program is designed for that type of bicycle.

< Means "less than."

Introduction to Aqua-Aerobics

Aqua-aerobics are exercises that you do while standing in a swimming pool or holding on to the sides of the pool. The main work occurs as a result of your pushing your limbs and trunk through the resistance of the water (see p. 73, "A Note on the Physics of Water Exercise").

These exercises can produce strength and aerobic conditioning. They are ideal for those with bone, joint, or muscle problems that are aggravated by activities done on land, against the force of gravity.

The first step is to warm up with some stretching exercises. Then, move on to the main aqua-aerobics workout. A graduated system of age-adjusted repetitions has also been included.

(*Note:* The source for all the following aqua-aerobics exercises and the accompanying illustrations is the *Aerobics* newsletter, copyright 1981, Institute for Aerobics Research.)

The Aqua-Aerobics Exercises

Stretching Exercise 1

1. Place your right foot flat against the pool wall.

2. Stretch forward, moving your upper body toward the knee. Keep the back straight and the chin up or bent slightly forward.

3. Hold for 10 to 20 seconds, then repeat for left leg.

This movement stretches the hamstrings, the calf muscles, and the lower back.

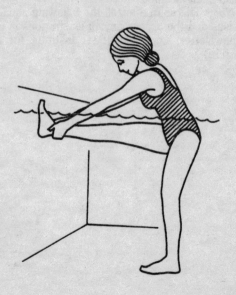

Stretching Exercise 2

1. Place both feet against the pool wall and hold on to the edge with both hands. Knees and elbows are bent. Hold for 10 to 20 seconds.

2. Slowly stretch out your legs while straightening your elbows and knees. Your feet should be flat against the wall. Hold for 10 to 20 seconds.

This exercise also stretches the hamstrings, the calf muscles, and the lower back.

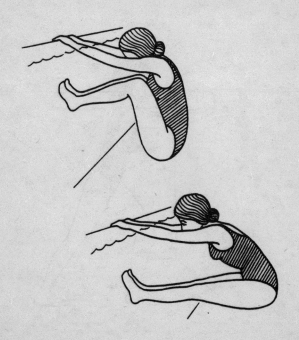

Stretching Exercise 3

1. Place your left foot 12 to 18 inches behind your right foot. Both hands should be flat against the pool wall, with toes pointing straight ahead.

2. Lean toward the pool wall, keeping your left knee straight and your left foot flat on the pool bottom.

3. Hold this position for 10 to 20 seconds, then repeat the movement for the right leg.

This exercise stretches the calf muscles and the Achilles tendon.

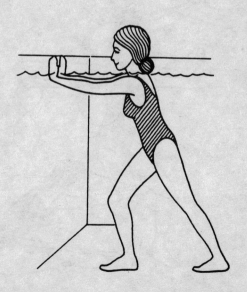

Arm Exercise 1

1. Place one foot in front of the other and bend your knees so that your shoulders are under water. Your arms should be held straight out to the sides, palms facing down.

2. With both arms working, inscribe figure 8s with your hands in the water. Keep your fingers together and your elbows and arms straight.

3. Begin with 10 repetitions, then follow the age-adjusted recommendations in the chart on p. 69.

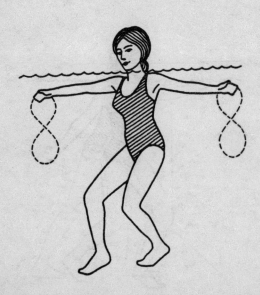

Arm Exercise 2

1. Place one foot in front of the other and bend your knees so that your shoulders are under water. Your arms should be held straight out in front of you, with palms facing down.

2. Swing your arms down by your sides and behind you, keeping your fingers together and your arms straight.

3. Rotate your arms so that the palms face forward and swing them back up. Throughout these motions, keep your arms completely under water.

4. Begin with 10 repetitions and then follow the age-adjusted recommendations in the chart on p. 69.

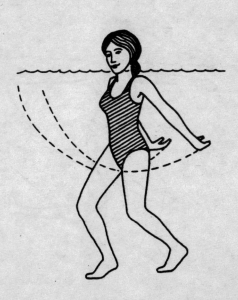

Thigh Exercise 1

1. Place your back against the pool wall and drape your arms along the pool edge to support your body. Your legs should be held straight out in front of your body, parallel to the bottom of the pool. Ankles should be flexed.

2. Pull your legs wide apart and then pull them back together.

3. Begin with 5 repetitions and then follow the age-adjusted recommendations in the chart on p. 69.

Note: Keep your stomach tucked in and press your lower back against the wall.

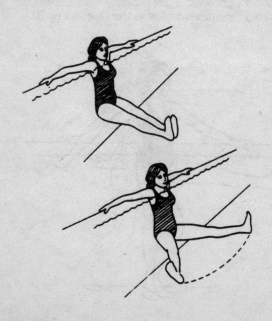

Thigh Exercise 2

1. Place your back against the pool wall in waist-deep water. Use both arms for support on the side of the pool. Stand on your left leg, with your right leg lifted straight up to the side. Your right ankle should be flexed.

2. Swing your right leg in front of your body and cross it over to your left side.

3. Swing your right leg back across your body and assume a standing position, with both feet on the bottom of the pool.

4. Repeat with left leg.

5. Begin with 5 repetitions, then follow the age-adjusted recommendations in the chart on p. 70.

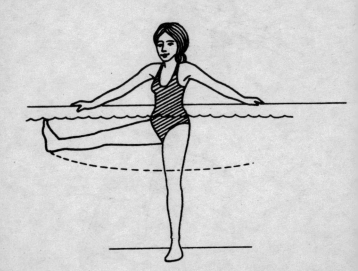

Thigh Exercise 3

1. Place your feet against the pool wall and hold on to the edge of the pool with both hands. Your knees and elbows should remain straight.

2. Push off with your feet and pull your legs apart into a straddle position. Your elbows will bend naturally as your body moves into the wall.

3. Push off with your feet again. Holding your legs straight, pull them together so that you return to the original position.

4. Begin with 5 repetitions and then follow the age-adjusted recommendations in the chart on p. 70.

Note: Remember to use your stomach muscles in executing these movements.

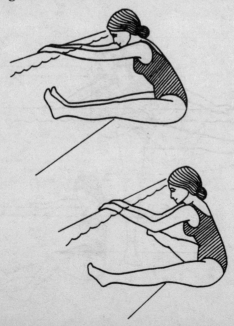

Waist and Stomach Exercise 1

1. Place your back against the pool wall and support your body by extending your arms along the edge of the pool. Your legs should be straight out in front of you, parallel to the bottom of the pool.

2. Keeping your back to the wall, swing both legs to the left side of the wall.

3. Contract your abdominal muscles and swing both legs across your body, toward the right side of the pool.

4. Begin with 8 repetitions (4 to the right and 4 to the left), then follow the age-adjusted recommendations in the chart on p. 70.

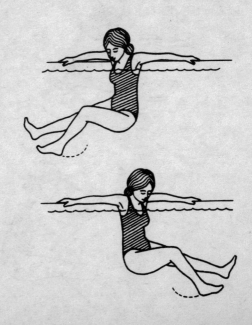

Waist and Stomach Exercise 2

1. Place your back toward the pool wall. Suspend your body from the edge by supporting yourself with both arms along the side of the pool. Allow your back to drift away from the wall.

2. Simultaneously pedal your legs as if you were riding a bike. Also, twist at the hips as you execute this movement. Alternate the twisting motion from the right side to the left. (I.e., as your right knee comes up toward your chest, rotate your hips to the left. Then, as the left leg comes up, rotate your hips to the right.)

Note: The bent knee is always on the top, and the legs are always under the water.

3. Begin with 20 pedaling motions (10 to the right and 10 to the left), then follow the age-adjusted recommendations in the chart on p. 70.

Waist and Stomach Exercise 3

1. Crouch so that your shoulders are under the water, with your knees bent and your weight on the balls of your feet.

2. Quickly rotate your hips back and forth, from right to left. Your arms will go in the opposite direction from your hips. During the twisting movement, your feet should leave the bottom of the pool.

3. Begin with 20 rotations (10 to the right and 10 to the left), and then follow the age-adjusted recommendations in the chart on p. 71.

Note: Hold your stomach in tightly throughout the exercise.

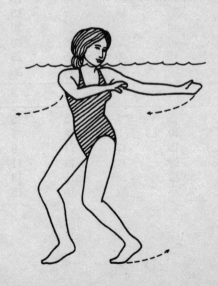

Aqua-Aerobics Stretching Exercises

| | *Repetitions* | | | | |
| | *Age (years)* | | | | |
Week	*<30*	*30–49*	*50–59*	*60+*	*Freq/wk*
	Arms 1				
1	10	10	10	10	3–4x
2	20	18	16	15	3–4x
3	30	25	22	20	3–4x
4	40	32	30	20	3–4x
5	45	40	35	25	3–4x
6	50	45	40	30	3–4x
	Arms 2				
1	10	10	10	10	3–4x
2	20	18	16	15	3–4x
3	30	25	22	20	3–4x
4	40	32	30	20	3–4x
5	45	40	35	25	3–4x
6	50	45	40	30	3–4x
	Thighs 1				
1	5	5	5	5	3–4x
2	10	9	8	7	3–4x
3	15	13	11	9	3–4x
4	20	17	14	11	3–4x
5	20	18	15	13	3–4x
6	25	22	18	15	3–4x

| | | Repetitions | | | |
| | | Age (years) | | | |
Week	<30	30–49	50–59	60 +	Freq/wk
Thighs 2					
1	15	5	5	5	3–4x
2	10	9	8	7	3–4x
3	15	13	11	9	3–4x
4	20	17	14	11	3–4x
5	20	18	15	13	3–4x
6	25	22	18	15	3–4x
Thighs 3					
1	5	5	5	5	3–4x
2	10	9	8	7	3–4x
3	15	13	11	9	3–4x
4	20	17	14	11	3–4x
5	20	18	15	13	3–4x
6	25	22	18	15	3–4x
Waist & Stomach 1					
1	8	8	8	8	3–4x
2	10	10	8	8	3–4x
3	12	12	10	10	3–4x
4	16	14	12	12	3–4x
5	20	18	16	14	3–4x
6	24	20	18	16	3–4x
Waist & Stomach 2					
1	20	20	20	20	3–4x
2	30	28	26	24	3–4x
3	40	36	32	28	3–4x
4	50	44	38	32	3–4x
5	60	52	44	36	3–4x
6	70	60	50	40	3–4x

Week	<30	30–49	50–59	60+	Freq/wk
			Repetitions		
			Age (years)		
		Waist & Stomach 3			
1	20	20	20	20	3–4x
2	30	28	26	24	3–4x
3	40	36	32	28	3–4x
4	50	44	38	32	3–4x
5	60	52	44	36	3–4x
6	70	60	50	40	3–4x

< Means "less than."

Source: *Aerobics Newsletter* © 1981, Institute for Aerobics Research.

Water Running and Walking

Water running and walking are not only good aerobic exercises but they are the only known ways to recover from a sports injury while improving performance. Exercise in water that is waist-deep and bring your knees up so that your feet are at least 6 to 8 inches off the bottom of the pool. Adjust the steps per minute to a pace that you can keep for the required time, age-adjusted. Exercise either in place or move around the pool. Remember: This type of exercise is a replacement for aqua-aerobics and is not expected to be done in conjunction with that type of exercise. However, 2 minutes of water running or walking is a good way to finish up an aqua-aerobics exercise class.

Water Running

Week	| Minutes				
	| Age (years)				
	30	30–49	50–59	60+	Freq/wk
1	2	2	2	1	3–4x
2	4	3	2	2	3–4x
3	6	5	4	3	3–4x
4	8	7	6	4	3–4x
5	10	9	8	6	3–4x
6	12	11	10	8	3–4x
7	14	13	12	10	3–4x
8	16	15	14	12	3–4x
9	18	17	16	14	3–4x
10	20	20	18	15	3–4x

Water Walking

Week	| Minutes				
	| Age (years)				
	30	30–49	50–59	60+	Freq/wk
1	5	5	5	5	3–4x
2	8	8	7	6	3–4x
3	10	9	8	7	3–4x
4	12	10	9	8	3–4x
5	15	14	12	10	3–4x
6	18	16	14	12	3–4x
7	20	18	16	14	3–4x
8	22	20	18	16	3–4x
9	24	22	20	18	3–4x
10	25	24	22	20	3–4x

A Note on the Physics of Water Exercise

The cardiovascular effects of exercise, whether on land or in the water, are fundamentally the same. But the *physics* underlying land and water exercises are quite different.

During water exercises such as swimming, the water supports from 93 to 100 percent of a swimmer's weight. As a result, an extremely obese person will expend little or no energy to stay afloat because fat floats in water. An extremely lean person, on the other hand, will expend considerably more energy to stay afloat. The reason: He can't float as easily because lean muscle tissue sinks in water, so he must tread water to stay afloat.

Another way to think of this is in terms of a person's loss of weight in water: An athletic, lean male, after completely exhaling, will usually weigh approximately 7 to 10 pounds when submerged in water. But an obese person under the same circumstances will be buoyant—that is, he will have *no* weight and will float.

With water exercises in which the participant is only partially submerged (e.g., water volleyball in a shallow pool), the water supports about half of the participant's body weight. A simple rule of thumb: Water roughly supports the percentage of the body submerged in it. So, a 150-pound male standing in water up to his navel would weigh about 75 pounds if he stood on a scale located at the bottom of the pool.

One difference between land exercises (e.g., running or walking) and water exercises (e.g., swimming or scuba diving) is that land activities generally test the body's ability to overcome gravity by forcing the individual to accelerate his mass against gravity. The role of air resistance (except on windy days) is usually negligible.

Water exercises, in contrast, primarily test the body's ability to move itself through a viscous resistance—i.e., water. Even though great effort may be required to move through the water, the work necessary to overcome gravity is generally negligible.

Half-submerged exercises seem to incorporate the best of the two worlds. The participant is forced to support some of his mass against gravity, though not as much as he would on land. He must also move half of his body through water, which is much more viscous than air.

In deeper water, the participant will face greater viscous water resistance and proportionately less impact to the skeletal system and joints. In shallow water, less viscous resistance is encountered, but there will be greater impact shocks to the body because of the greater influence of gravity.

The implications of water exercises for those with joint, skeletal, or muscle problems that are aggravated by gravity are obvious: Cardiovascular fitness is possible without the high risk of injury or discomfort that may accompany land exercises such as running or jogging.

4

Control Through Diet

What should be the role of diet in controlling hypertension?

Lawrence Beilin, in his "State of the Art Lecture" published in the Australian *Journal of Hypertension*, sums up the current understanding:

"There is now substantial evidence to suggest that diet, physical inactivity and alcohol consumption are the three major environmental influences on blood pressure levels. . . ."

Many hypertensives, especially those with mild forms of the disease, have gained *complete* control over their blood pressure through dietary means. But even if diet alone won't do the job for you, a wise food plan, combined with other pressure-lowering treatments such as exercise and/or medications, is an essential ingredient in *any* treatment strategy.

An effective meal plan will meet the challenge of high blood pressure—and the risk factors associated with hypertension—in a number of ways:

> *Principle 1. Stay at your ideal weight.* The plan should reduce excess weight, or promote the maintenance of one's ideal weight. A major objective is to eliminate upper-body fat (at the waist and

above), which is an important risk factor for hypertension.

Because there are no known techniques for spot reducing, the goal should be to get rid of excess weight *throughout* the body. This approach will automatically cut down on upper-body fat.

Principle 2. Take in plenty of potassium. The menus should be high in potassium, especially for those on a diuretic medication that causes the loss of potassium through excessive urination.

Your diet should contain an extra 1,000 to 2,000 mg of potassium over and above the normal requirement, or a total of approximately 4,000 to 5,000 mg daily. Usually, six to eight high-potassium foods will meet this goal.

The following charts may be used as a guide to ensure that your diet provides adequate potassium to replace any urinary losses. *Note:* Many of these foods have been included in the Menu and Recipe sections of the Antihypertensive Meal Plan presented later in this chapter.

High-Potassium Foods

The following list of foods high in potassium may be used as a guide to ensure that your diet contains adequate potassium to replace urinary losses. Plan your diet to contain an extra 1,000 to 2,000 mg of potassium daily (for a total of 4–5,000 mg daily) if you have a potassium deficiency or are undergoing chronic therapy with diuretics. Usually, six to eight high-potassium foods will meet this goal.

Fruits	Serving Size	Approximate Potassium Content (mg)
Apricots	3 medium	280
Avocado	½	680
Banana	1 medium	440
Cantaloupe	½ melon	800
Dates	10 pieces	520
Grapefruit	1 cup, or 1 large	260
Honeydew melon	⅛ melon	210
Orange	1 medium	270
Prunes, dried	5 pieces	350
Raisins	2 tablespoons	140
Strawberries, fresh	1 cup	250
Watermelon	1 cup	160

Juices and Milk		
Grapefruit juice	1 cup	400
Milk	1 cup	370
Orange juice	1 cup	500
Pineapple juice	1 cup	380
Prune juice	1 cup	600
Tomato juice	1 cup	540

Vegetables		
Artichoke	1 medium	360
Broccoli, cooked	½ cup	200
Brussels sprouts cooked	½ cup	230
Carrots, cooked	½ cup	160
Dried beans	½ cup	420
Greens, cooked	½ cup	160
Lima beans, cooked	½ cup	360
Potato, baked	2½-inch	450
Spinach, cooked	½ cup	300

Vegetables	Serving Size	Approximate Potassium Content (mg)
Squash, winter	½ cup	470
Sweet potato, baked	1 small	340
Tomato, raw	1 medium	300

Meats and Nuts		
Beef	3 ounces	200–300
Fish	3 ounces	350–500
Hamburger	3 ounces	200–250
Turkey & chicken	3 ounces	200–350
Peanuts	3½ ounces	630

Miscellaneous

Bran cereal, wheat germ, whole-grain breads and cereals, peanut butter, chocolate, catsup, dried parsley, instant tea or coffee or Postum, salt substitute (with physician's consent).

> *Principle 3. Limit sodium.* A diet to control hypertension should limit sodium intake significantly—preferably keeping the consumption at a level of about 2 grams (2,000 mg) per day. The following suggestions should give you some ideas about how to achieve this goal.

More on Sodium Management

The average person should be eating about 1,100 to 3,300 mg of sodium per day, according to the Food and Nutrition Board of the National Academy of Sciences. For hypertensives or those at risk for high blood pressure, I recommend 2,000 mg or less daily.

Despite these recommendations, however, the typical American *actually* averages about 3,000 to 5,850 mg of sodium per day! Remember: Salt is composed of approximately 40 percent sodium and 60 percent chloride. So if a person is consuming 4,000 mg of sodium daily, he's taking in 10,000 mg of salt!

Where does all this sodium come from? The following chart, printed in *Environmental Nutrition* (March 1988) and adapted from the National Dairy Council's *Contemporary Topics in Nutrition*, should give you an idea:

Sources of Dietary Sodium

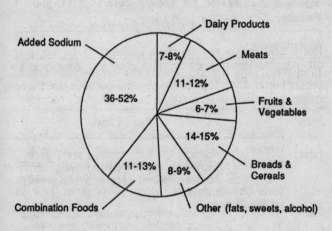

Note: According to other authoritative reports, the "added sodium" category comprises less than one-third of the total, and greater amounts come from various processed foods. (See Fregly, "Estimates of Sodium and Potassium Intake.")

• • •

Salt seems to confront us at every turn as we attempt to plan a restrictive diet. However, plenty of low-sodium strategies are available. Following are some practical suggestions about how to limit your daily sodium intake:

Sodium suggestion 1. First, reduce the salt in your cooking to half the amount you would normally use. Then, gradually cut salt completely, and add more herbs and spices. The following chart can help you create your own herb-and-spice flavors.

How to Cook with Herbs and Spices

Herbs and spices are excellent alternatives to salt and other high-sodium products. This chart can guide you in creating your own flavors.

Food	Season with—
Beef	allspice, bay leaf, caraway seed, garlic, marjoram, dry mustard, nutmeg, onion, broiled peaches, pepper, green pepper, thyme
Fish	bay leaf, curry, marjoram, dry mustard, lemon, parsley, margarine, lemon juice, green pepper, tomatoes
Lamb	basil, curry, garlic powder, mint, rosemary, thyme
Poultry	cranberries, parsley, paprika, rosemary, sage, thyme
Veal	bay leaf, curry, ginger, marjoram, oregano, rosemary, thyme
Eggs	curry, dry mustard, onion, paprika, parsley, thyme, green pepper, tomatoes

Food	Season with—
Asparagus	caraway seed, lemon juice, mustard seed, sesame seed, tarragon
Beans	basil, dill seed, unsalted French dressing, lemon juice, marjoram, mint, mustard seed, nutmeg, oregano, sage, savory, tarragon, thyme
Beets	allspice, bay leaves, caraway seed, cloves, dill seed, mustard seed, tarragon
Broccoli	caraway seed, dill seed, mustard seed, oregano, tarragon
Cabbage	caraway seed, dill seed, mint, mustard seed, dry mustard, nutmeg, poppy seed, savory, thyme, vinegar
Cauliflower	caraway seed, chives, dill seed, lemon juice, mace, nutmeg, parsley, rosemary, tarragon
Corn	curry, green pepper
Cucumbers	basil, dill seed, lemon juice, mint, tarragon, nutmeg
Eggplant	chives, grated onion or garlic, marjoram, oregano, chopped parsley, tarragon
Lettuce salad	basil, caraway seed, chives, dill, garlic, lemon, onion, tarragon, thyme, vinegar
Onions	caraway seed, mustard seed, nutmeg, oregano, pepper, sage, thyme
Peas	basil, dill, marjoram, mint, oregano, lemon, parsley, green pepper, poppy seed, rosemary, sage, savory, thyme
Potatoes	basil, bay leaves, caraway seed, chives, dill seed, mace, mustard seed, onion, oregano, paprika, parsley, green pepper, poppy seed, rosemary, thyme

Food	Season with—
Spinach	basil, mace, marjoram, nutmeg, oregano
Squash	allspice, basil, cinnamon, chives, cloves, fennel, ginger, mace, mustard seed, nutmeg, onion, rosemary
Sweet potatoes	allspice, cardamon, cinnamon, cloves, nutmeg
Tomatoes	allspice, basil, bay leaf, curry, marjoram, onion, sage, thyme

- When experimenting with herbs and spices, add small amounts at a time, ¼ teaspoon of dried herbs for every 4 servings of food.

- Fresh herbs can be substituted for dried herbs: ⅓ teaspoon ground herbs = 1 teaspoon dried herbs = 1 tablespoon fresh herbs.

- One average-size fresh garlic clove = ⅛ teaspoon dehydrated powder, minced, or chopped garlic.

- Leaf herbs should be crushed before adding to recipes to release more flavor.

- Use pure herbs and spices instead of seasoned salt (onion and garlic powder—*not* onion and garlic salt).

- Whole spices such as stick cinnamon and cloves can enhance the flavor of beverages. Ground spices can "cloud" the liquid.

- Whole spices should be added at the beginning of the cooking process. Ground spices should be added toward the end, since their flavors are quickly released in hot foods.

- Herbs and spices should be stored in a cool, dry, dark place (not over the kitchen stove). They have a six-month shelf life; they can be frozen in plastic bags.

- Prepare your own salt-free blends to use in cooking and in the salt shaker at your table.

1. Season-All (mix for meats and vegetables)

1 teaspoon basil	1 teaspoon mace
1 teaspoon marjoram	1 teaspoon ground cloves
1 teaspoon thyme	¼ teaspoon nutmeg
1 teaspoon oregano	1 teaspoon black pepper
1 teaspoon parsley	¼ teaspoon cayenne
1 teaspoon savory	

2. All-Purpose Spice Blend

5 teaspoons onion powder	2½ teaspoons mustard powder
2½ teaspoons paprika	½ teaspoon ground white pepper
1¼ teaspoons thyme	
¼ teaspoon celery seed	
2½ teaspoons garlic powder	

3. Herbed Seasoning Blend

2 tablespoons dill weed or basil	¼ teaspoon grated lemon peel (dried)
1 teaspoon oregano leaves, crushed	1 teaspoon celery seed
2 tablespoons onion powder	⅟₁₆ teaspoon black pepper

4. Spicy Flavor Blend

2 tablespoons savory, crushed	1¼ teaspoons ground white pepper
2½ teaspoons onion powder	½ teaspoon garlic powder
1⅜ teaspoons curry powder	
1¼ teaspoons cumin	
1 tablespoon powdered mustard	

Sodium suggestion 2. Avoid adding salt to your foods after cooking has been completed, or at the dinner table.

Sodium suggestion 3. Use oil and vinegar in place of commercial salad dressings, which are high in sodium. Or, reduce the sodium in bottled dressing by diluting it with an equal amount of water and vinegar.

Sodium suggestion 4. Substitute one tablespoon of vinegar (no sodium) mixed with one cup of skim milk (125 mg sodium) for one cup of buttermilk (318 mg sodium).

Sodium suggestion 5. Substitute the following recipes for canned tomato products:

- One can of salt-free tomato paste *plus* 1 can of cold water *equals* salt-free tomato puree.

- One can of salt-free tomato paste *plus* 2 cans of cold water *equals* salt-free tomato sauce.

- One can of salt-free tomato paste *plus* 3 cans of cold water *plus* lemon juice *plus* tabasco sauce *equals* salt-free tomato juice.

- One can of salt-free tomato paste *plus* 2 cans of cold water *plus* 2 tablespoons of apple cider *plus* 1½ tablespoons of frozen pineapple-juice concentrate *equals* salt-free catsup.

Sodium suggestion 6. Substitute low-sodium ("lite") soy sauce for regular soy sauce, or dilute regular soy sauce with an equal part of water.

Sodium suggestion 7. Make your own low-sodium bouillon cubes: Freeze low-sodium chicken broth in a miniature ice tray. Then, pop cubes out and store them in the freezer for later use.

Sodium suggestion 8. Read food labels closely. Many reduced-sodium products are available. The Food and Drug Administration has established these label criteria:

- "No sodium" or "sodium-free": less than 5 mg of sodium per serving

- "Very low-sodium": 35 mg of sodium or less per serving

- "Low-sodium": 140 mg of sodium or less per serving

- "Reduced sodium": sodium content reduced by 75 percent as compared with similar products prepared with salt

- "Unsalted": food product that is normally salted has been processed without salt.

Sodium suggestion 9. Prepare your own marinade recipes as follows:

- *For fish:*
  1 teaspoon tarragon
  1 tablespoon lemon juice
  1 teaspoon low-sodium soy sauce
  freshly ground pepper to taste

- *For poultry:*
  1 small minced onion
  1 minced garlic clove
  ¼ cup low-sodium catsup
  ¼ cup low-sodium soy sauce
  1 cup white wine
  1½ tablespoons brown sugar
  freshly ground pepper to taste

- *For turkey:*
  ½ cup Kitchen Bouquet (a liquid seasoning blend)
    generously rubbed over turkey
  1 small chopped onion
  4 sliced celery stalks
  6 tablespoons garlic powder
  6 tablespoons onion powder
  2 to 3 tablespoons freshly ground pepper

Sodium suggestion 10. Limit or eliminate such high-sodium foods as these:

Salty or smoked meats—ham, bacon, luncheon meats, hot dogs, sausage, chipped or corned beef, salt pork.

Salty or smoked fish—anchovies, caviar, herring, sardines. *Note:* choose tuna packed in water or "reduced sodium" brands.

Processed cheeses or cheese products. Look for "natural" cheese on the label.

Consommé, canned soups (unless low-sodium), dried soup mixes.

Canned vegetables or vegetable juice (unless low-sodium), sauerkraut, pork and beans.

Snack foods—potato chips, pretzels, salted nuts, salted popcorn, snack crackers, party dips and spreads, crackers with salted toppings.

Olives, pickles, relishes, bottled salad dressings (unless low-sodium).

Meat extracts and tenderizers.

Prepared sauces—barbecue, chili, steak, soy, tomato, tartar, worcestershire, mustard, catsup.

Condiments—spices containing salt or MSG (monosodium glutamate), lemon pepper.

Other foods—frozen dinners, instant cereals, instant pudding mixes, pizza, fast foods, pot pies.

Breakfast cereals, except for those *lowest* in sodium. (The lowest-sodium cereals include shredded wheat, puffed wheat, puffed rice, low-sodium corn flakes, low-sodium Rice Krispies.)

Sodium suggestion 11. Check your medicines. They often contain salt (e.g., Alka-Seltzer, various antacids such as Rolaids, Metamucil instant mix, Vick's cough medicines, laxatives, pain relievers, and sedatives).

Sodium suggestion 12. Use available unsalted or low-sodium commercial products. (See the following list.)

Some Currently Available Unsalted or Low-Sodium Products

Condiments

Unsalted margarine
Unsalted diet margarine
Unsalted mayonnaise
Unsalted salad dressings
Unsalted catsup
Lite soy sauce

Salt-free seasonings
  see "How to Cook with
  Herbs and Spices," p. 234)
Low-sodium canned broth
Low-sodium bouillon cubes

Protein

Low-sodium tuna,
  packed in water
Low-sodium peanut butter

Low-sodium cheeses
Low-sodium cottage cheese

Snacks

Unsalted rice cakes
Unsalted popcorn
Unsalted melba toast
Crackers with unsalted tops

Low-sodium crackers
Unsalted nuts
Unsalted pretzels
Unsalted chips

Vegetables

Low-sodium canned soups
Low-sodium canned
  vegetables
Low-sodium tomato sauce

Low-sodium spaghetti sauce
Low-sodium tomato juice
Low-sodium V-8 juice
Low-sodium pickles

Sodium suggestion 13. Use commercial seasoning alternatives to sodium. (See the following list.)

Low-Sodium Commercial
Seasoning Products

- *Salt substitutes* taste like salt but contain little or no sodium. These products usually contain potassium chloride (KCl) and should be used as directed by a physician or dietitian and are unadvisable for kidney patients:
  Salt substitutes containing potassium chloride:
    Morton Salt Substitute
    Estee Salt-It Salt Substitute
    Estee Salt-It Seasoning
    Kroger Seasoned Salt Substitute
- *Commercial Low-Sodium Seasonings:*
  Lawry's Seasoned Pepper
          Salt-Free 17 Seasoning
          Natural Choice
          Seasoned Salt-Free
  Adolph's Unsalted 100% Natural Tenderizer
  McCormick Chinese Five Spice
             Italian Seasoning
             Salt-Free Parsley Patch Lemon Pepper
             Salt-Free Parsley Patch All-Purpose Seasoning
             Salt-Free Parsley Patch Popcorn Blend
             Salt-Free Parsley Patch Sesame All-Purpose Seasoning
             Salt-Free Parsley Patch Garlic Salt-less
             Salt-Free Parsley Patch It's A Dilly
  Norcliff Thayer, Inc. Seasoned No Salt
  Mrs. Dash Lemon and Herb Salt-Free
            Extra Spice
            Original Blend
            Low Pepper No Garlic
  Kroger Italian Seasoning
  Future Foods, Inc. Salt-Free Enhance—All-Purpose Seasoning
  Jane's Krazy Mixed-Up Pepper
  Estee Salt-Free Seasoning Sense All-Purpose Spice Blend
         Salt-Free Seasoning Sense Mexican Spice Blend
         Salt-Free Seasoning Sense Oriental Spice Blend
  Voyager Captain's Table All-Purpose Seasoning

Spice Islands No-Salt All-Purpose Seasoning
- *Commercial Low-Sodium Liquid Seasonings:*
  Kikkoman Low-Sodium Soy Sauce
  Angostura Aromatic Bitters
  Kitchen Bouquet
  Wyler's Low-Sodium Bouillon Cubes
  Featherweight Low-Sodium Bouillon Granules
  Tabasco Sauce
  Hot Pepper Sauce
  Low-Sodium V-8 Juice
- *Other Seasoning Suggestions:*
  Horseradish
  Orange or lemon zest—shredded colored part of the peel
  (with discarded white bitter layer)

Sodium suggestion 14. Choose "natural" or unprocessed foods over processed foods whenever possible. As a general rule, the sodium content of food increases as food processing increases.

To learn more about the sodium content of various seasonings and foods, consider the following chart:

Sodium Comparisons

Note: Sodium content increases as food processing increases.

Food	Amount	Sodium (mg)
Apple	1 medium	1
Applesauce	1 cup	6
Apple pie	⅛ pie, frozen	482
Bread	1 slice	130
Homemade biscuit	1 biscuit	175
Canned biscuit	1 biscuit	270
Butter	1 tablespoon, unsalted	2
Butter	1 tablespoon, salted	120
Margarine	1 tablespoon	150
Cabbage	1 cup	22
Cole slaw	1 cup	150
Sauerkraut	1 cup, canned	1,760

Food	Amount	Sodium (mg)
Chicken	3 ounces, baked	86
Fast-food chicken	3 ounces, fried	500
Chicken pie	1 pie, frozen	863
Corn	1 ear	1
Corn flakes	1 cup	325
Canned kernels	1 cup	400
Lemon	1 lemon	3
Soy sauce	1 tablespoon	1,330
Salt	1 teaspoon	2,130
Peanuts without salt	1 ounce (30 nuts)	1
Peanut butter	1 tablespoon	95
Peanuts with salt	1 ounce (30 nuts)	120
Cheese, cheddar	1 ounce	175
Cheese spread	1 ounce	380
Cheese soup	1 cup, canned	1,020
Pork chop	3 ounces, baked	54
Bacon	3 pieces	303
Sausage	1 patty	418
Baked potato	1 medium	5
French fries	½ cup (18 fries)	120
Potato chips	½ cup (10 chips)	200
Tomato	1 medium	4
Tomato juice	1 cup	500
Tomato sauce	1 cup (Del Monte)	1,300
Tomato paste	1 cup (Del Monte)	60
Tomato soup	1 cup, canned	970
Spaghetti sauce	1 cup	2,000
Tuna in water	3 ounces	372
Tuna in oil	3 ounces	442
Tuna noodle casserole	1 cup	715
Water	12 ounces, tap	4
Soft drink	12 ounces	30–60
Club soda	12 ounces	90

Printed with permission from *The Balancing Act* by G. Kostas and K. Rojohn, © 1989.

Low-Sodium Strategies
for Eating Out

As conscientious and disciplined as a person may be in preparing and eating low-sodium dishes, the best of intentions may fall by the wayside at a restaurant. As a result, it's *essential* for those on a low-sodium diet to devise and strictly adhere to eating strategies that will keep their consumption of sodium as low as possible. Following are a few general guidelines:

- When you order in a restaurant, choose simply prepared dishes, such as grilled meat, a baked potato, or a tossed salad with oil and vinegar dressing. Avoid casseroles and combination dishes of unknown (and probably sodium-rich) ingredients.

- Request that dishes be prepared without added salt, monosodium glutamate (MSG), or sauces.

- Request that dishes be prepared with lemon juice instead of salt.

- When you travel by air, request low-sodium meals or fresh fruit plates at least twenty-four hours in advance of your departure (or earlier if the airline requires more notice).

In addition, it's important for those committed to a low-sodium diet to know what to do about fast food meals. To this end, consult the "Tips on Ordering at a Fast Food Restaurant" (below) and the "Nutritional Values of Certain Lower Sodium Fast Food Meals" (p. 93). A more complete listing of the nutritional values of fast foods is in appendix III.

Tips on Ordering at
a Fast Food Restaurant

1. Dine defensively: Choose items that aren't excessive in fat, sodium, or calories. Balance your fast food meal with a nutritious breakfast and dinner that include fewer fat calories, more fruit, more vegetables, and lower-fat dairy products than you normally eat.

2. Choose roast beef sandwiches instead of burgers.

3. Choose a small, plain burger instead of a larger, deluxe hamburger, or split a sandwich with a friend.

4. Omit mayonnaise (1 tablespoon = 100 calories) and cheese (1 ounce = 100 calories) from your sandwich. Instead, order lettuce, tomato, and onion (1 slice = 20 calories).

5. In place of a traditional burger, choose a baked potato and salad. Dressing suggestions: low-calorie dressings, lemon juice, picante sauce, or a small amount of cottage cheese.

6. Limit fried foods. Calories are almost triple in deep-fried items. Fat can be reduced significantly by removing the crust before eating (i.e., on fried chicken). Also, choose "regular" fried instead of "extra crispy."

7. Skip French fries, or split an order, or choose a baked potato instead.

8. Limit desserts, sweets, milkshakes, pies, and ice cream, or carry a piece of fruit from home to add to your meal.

9. Salad bars: eat carrots, tomatoes, cucumbers, mushrooms, green peppers, lettuce, and dark green vegetables, as desired. Limit dressings, croutons, pasta, potato-type salads, cheeses, nuts, and seeds. For dressings, use oil and vinegar, flavored vinegar, fresh squeezed

lemon, or low-calorie varieties. Some packets of regular salad dressing contain more than 300 calories and in excess of 300 mg of sodium. Also, they may have more fat than a large burger!

10. Pizza: Order cheese pizza with green peppers, onions, and mushrooms. Limit servings to 1 to 2 pieces, and order a dinner salad. *Note:* This meal contains about 1,000 mg of sodium—half a day's allowance for those on a low-sodium diet!

11. Omit pickles, mustard, catsup, special sauces, cheese, processed meats (such as bacon, ham, sausage, hot dogs, pepperoni, and salami), anchovies, and olives.

Nutritional Values of Lower Sodium Fast Food Meals

	Calories	Fat (g)	Cholesterol (mg)	Sodium (mg)
McDonald's				
Chicken Salad Oriental	146	4	92	270
Lite vinaigrette dressing (½ packet)	25	1	1	150
2% Milk (8 ounces)	121	5	5	145
Fresh fruit (from home)	80	0	0	0
Total	372	10	98	565
Burger King				
Hamburger	275	12	37	509
Side salad	20	0	0	10
Reduced-calorie Italian dressing (½ packet)	7	0	0	213
2% Milk (8 ounces)	121	5	5	145
Total	423	17	42	877

	Calories	Fat (g)	Cholesterol (mg)	Sodium (mg)
Arby's				
Regular Roast Beef Sandwich	353	15	39	588
Fresh fruit (from home)	80	0	0	0
Total	433	15	39	588
Jack-in-the-Box				
Chicken Fajita Pita	292	8	34	703
Side salad	51	3	0	84
Reduced-calorie French dressing (½ packet)	40	2	0	150
Total	383	13	34	937
Wendy's				
Chicken Sandwich/ no mayonnaise	340	12	60	565
½ Baked potato	125	1	0	30
Total	465	13	60	595
Or: Baked potato with	250	2	0	60
¼ cup cottage cheese	55	2	10	213
or 2 tablespoons grated imitation cheddar cheese	40	3	N/A	155
or 2 tablespoons grated Parmesan cheese	50	5	0	255
or taco sauce (1 packet)	10	0	0	105
or chives, mushrooms, green onions (use as desired)	0	0	0	0
Total	250–315	2–7	0–10	60–315

With these principles in mind, let's move on to the meal plans designed to prevent or treat hypertension. The first step in using the menus requires an understanding of the food exchange system, which will give you greater flexibility in departing from the listed menus and meals and in building your own personal diet program.

Understanding the
Food Exchange System

Some people prefer to follow our menus exactly as they are presented. But many may want to experiment with different foods, substituting here and eliminating there, and thus injecting more variety into the plan.

To this end, our menus have been set up according to the food exchange system. This concept is based on the principle that certain foods are interchangeable with others so that dieters can choose what they want to eat on a given day.

For an exchange system to work properly, similar foods must be grouped together according to their content of carbohydrate, protein, and fat. All the choices on each exchange list are roughly equal in calories. With these comparable groupings, any food on a list can be exchanged for any other food on the same list.

For example, as you examine the menus, you'll see that the food exchange category is listed after each food item. So (Milk) refers to milk products, and (Meat) refers to various types of protein-rich foods, such as fish, poultry, and beans.

More specifically, the exchange groups include the following categories:

1. Milk and milk products—protein sources

2. Meat and substitutes—protein sources

3. Bread/starches—complex carbohydrate sources

4. Vegetables—complex carbohydrate sources

5. Fruits—complex carbohydrate sources

6. Fats—fat sources

Note: When I use the term *complex carbohydrates*, I'm referring to foods that don't just contain simple sugars but instead provide a relatively wide range of nutrients, in addition to their sugar content.

With this information at your fingertips, feel free to substitute (i.e, "exchange") one type of milk product for another, or one type of meat for another, *provided* that the portions are the same, as indicated in the exchange tables.

Caution: If the portion size varies, so will the calories and nutrients. On the other hand, if the food types and portion sizes stay constant, you can vary the menus, while keeping comparable calorie and nutrient levels.

Finally, a word about the way the diets are balanced: Any well-constructed diet must include the basic nutrients of carbohydrate, protein, and fat. In our menus, these nutrients are available in the following percentages each day:

- Carbohydrates—50 to 70 percent of total calories

- Protein—10 to 20 percent of total calories

- Fat—20 to 30 percent of total calories

Using the exchange system will provide you with a variety of food choices and ensure a good balance of carbohydrate, protein, and fat throughout the day. In addition, you'll get an excellent mix of vitamins and minerals.

Following is a detailed listing of the food exchanges in each of the main categories. I've also included some tips on preparing meats, and on identifying specific portions of foods for purposes of the exchange system.

Protein

Milk & Milk Products
One serving contains 80 calories
(8 grams protein, 12 grams carbohydrate)

Eat

Milk (nonfat, skim, ½%, 1%)	1 cup
evaporated	½ cup
powdered	¼ cup
Low-fat 2% milk	¼ cup
Buttermilk (made from nonfat milk)[4]	1 cup
Yogurt	
from skim milk, plain, unflavored	1 cup
from low-fat milk, plain, unflavored	½ cup
Low-calorie hot cocoa or milkshake	
(i.e., Alba, Swiss Miss, Carnation, etc.)	1 cup

Avoid

Whole milk products:	Instant breakfast drinks[4]
chocolate	Flavored yogurts
condensed	Eggnog
dried	Ice cream
evaporated	Custard
Buttermilk (made from whole milk)[4]	Pudding
Flavored milk drink mixes[4]	

[4]–high in salt (sodium)

Protein

Meat/Substitutes
One serving (1 ounce) contains 70 calories
(8 grams protein, 3–5 grams fat)
Eat 4–8 ounces meat or substitutes daily

Eat

Choose 10 + meals per week:

Poultry (without skin)	
chicken, turkey, cornish hen, squab	1 ounce
Fish—any kind (fresh or frozen)	1 ounce
water-packed tuna or salmon, crab or lobster[4]	¼ cup
clams, oysters, scallops, shrimp	1 ounce or 5
sardines, drained[4]	3
Veal—any lean cut	1 ounce
Peanut butter[4], not hydrogenated (read labels)	1 tablespoon
Dried beans, peas (count as 1 meat + 1 bread)	½ cup
Chicken or turkey cold cuts[4]	
turkey ham, turkey bologna	1 ounce

Limit to 4 meals per week:

Lean beef cuts	
tenderloin (sirloin, filet, T-bone, porterhouse), round, cube, flank	1 ounce
roasts, stews—sirloin tip, round rump, chuck, arm	1 ounce
other—ground round or (chuck 15% fat ground beef), chipped beef, venison	1 ounce
Lean lamb cuts—leg, chops, loin, shoulder	1 ounce
Lean pork and ham[4]	
center cut steaks, loin chops, smoked ham[4]	1 ounce

Limit to 3 to 5 ounces per week:

Cholesterol-free cheese[4]

   Cheezola, Countdown, Kraft
     "Golden Image," etc.   1 ounce

Low-fat cheese[4]

   low-fat cottage cheese, Laughing Cow,
     farmer's, skim ricotta   1 ounce or ¼ cup

Medium-fat cheese[4]

   Bonbel, mozzarella, Parmesan, neufchatel   1 ounce or ¼ cup

Limit to 1 to 3 egg yolks per week:

Whole egg   1

Egg substitutes[4] (cholesterol-free)   ¼ cup

Egg whites   as desired

Limit to one 3-ounce serving per month:

Organ meats—liver, heart, brains, kidney

Avoid

Poultry—duck, goose, poultry skin

Fish—fish row (caviar); limit shrimp

Meats—fried, with gravies, sauces, breading, casseroles
       high fat meats:
         beef—brisket, corned beef, ground hamburger, club or rib
            steaks, rib roasts, spare ribs
         pork—bacon[4], deviled ham[4], loin, spare ribs, sausage[4], cold
            cuts[4]
         pork—hot dogs[4], luncheon meats[4]

Cheese[4]—all except skim milk or cholesterol-free cheese (see
       above)

Convenience foods—canned[4] or frozen meats, cream cheese,
cheese spreads[4], dips[4], packaged dinners[4], pork and beans[4], pizza[4],
fast foods[4], cold cuts[4].

[4]–high in salt (sodium)

Carbohydrate

Starches
One serving contains 70 calories
(2 grams of protein, 15 grams of carbohydrate)

Eat	
Bread and substitutes:	
Bread, any type	1 slice
Bread, "extra thin" (30 calories/slice)	2 slices
Bread crumbs	3 tablespoons
Bagel, small	½
Biscuit (2" across, made with proper fat)	1
Cornbread, 1½" cube	1
English muffin	½
Hamburger or hot dog bun	½
Pita or pocket bread	½
Rice cakes	2
Roll, plain soft	1
Tortilla (6" diameter, made without lard)	1
Cereal and cereal products:	
Bran cereals	½ cup
Dry cereal (flaked)	¼ cup
Dry cereal (puffed)	1 cup
Grapenuts	¼ cup
Cooked cereal (oatmeal, etc.)	½ cup
Cooked grits, noodles, rice, spaghetti	½ cup
Popcorn (popped, no fat added)	3 cups
Wheat germ or bran	¼ cup
Starchy Vegetables:	
Corn	½ cup
Corn-on-the-cob (3" long)	1 small
Mixed vegetables	½ cup
Lima Beans	½ cup
Parsnips	½ cup
Peas, green[4] (canned or frozen)	½ cup
Potato, white	1 small
Potato, mashed	½ cup
Pumpkin[2]	¼ cup

[4]–high in salt (sodium)
[2]–high in Vitamin A

Winter squash (acorn or butternut)[2]	½ cup
Yam or sweet potato[2]	¼ cup

Crackers:

Animal	10
Arrowroot	3
Bread sticks (4" x ¼")	2
Graham, 2½" square	2
Hollund rusks	1½
Matzoth, 4" x 6"	½
Melba Toast	4
Oyster (½ cup)[4]	20
Pretzels, 3⅛" x ⅛"[4]	25
Pretzels (unsalted small circles)	10
Rye Wafers, 2" x 3½"	3
Rye Krisp[4]	3
Saltines 2" square[4]	6
Soda, 2½" square[4]	4

Dried beans and Lentils:

Beans, Peas, Lentils dried and cooked (½ cup = 1 meat + 1 starch)	½ cup
Baked beans, no pork (if canned)[4]	¼ cup
Chickpeas, garbanzo beans	¼ cup

Miscellaneous:

Catsup, chili sauce or BBQ sauce[4]	¼ cup
Tomato sauce[4]	½ cup
Cornmeal, cornstarch, flour	2 tablespoons
Cornflake crumbs	3 tablespoons

Soups: 1 cup

Broth or tomato-based
(i.e., vegetable, chicken noodle)[4]
Homemade, with allowed ingredients
Canned soup[4]—refrigerate and remove
hardened fat
Fat-free broth or consommé—eat as desired

[2]–high in Vitamin A
[4]–high in salt (sodium)

Avoid

Butter rolls	Doughnuts[4]
Cereals, sugar-coated	Egg & cheese bread
Coffee cake[4]	Fried foods
Commercial baked goods	Granola cereals
Commercial popcorn[4]	unless homemade
Cornbread, biscuit, bread,	Pancakes, waffles[4]
cake mixes[4]	Pastries[4]
Crackers, flavored[4]	Potato chips[4]
Cream soup[4]	Sweet rolls[4]
Croissants	

Note: Read food labels carefully to avoid foods with undesirable fats and sodium.

[4]–high in salt (sodium)

Carbohydrate

Fruit/Juice
One serving contains 40 calories
(10 grams of carbohydrates)
Count one large fruit as 2 portions (80 calories)

Eat

Fresh, frozen, or canned fruit or fruit juice without sugar or syrup; cranberries can be used as desired if no sugar is added.

Apple	½ (4″ diameter) or 1 (2″ diameter)
Applesauce	½ cup
Apricots[2]	2 fresh
Apricots, dried[2]	4 halves
Banana	½ (3″ long)
Berries:	
Blackberries	½ cup
Blueberries	½ cup
Boysenberries	½ cup
Raspberries	½ cup
Strawberries[1]	¾ cup

[1]–high in Vitamin C
[2]–high in Vitamin A

Cherries	10 large
Dates	2
Figs, fresh or dried	1
Fruit cocktail	½ cup
Grapefruit[1]	½
sections	½ cup
Grapes	12 large
Kiwi	½
Mango[1]	½ small
Melon:	
Cantaloupe[3]	¼ (6″ diameter)
Casaba[2]	¼ (6″ diameter)
Honeydew[1]	⅛ (7″ diameter)
Watermelon[2]	1 cup
Melon balls[3]	¾ cup
Nectarine	1 small
Orange[1]	1 small
Orange sections[1]	½ small
Papaya[3]	¾ cup
Peach, fresh[2]	1 medium
Pear, fresh	1 small
Pear, canned	2 halves
Pineapple, diced	½ cup
Pineapple, sliced	1½ slices
Plums	2 medium
Prunes, dried	2 medium
Raisins	2 tablespoons
Tangerine[1]	1 medium

Juices

Apple juice	⅓ cup
Cider	⅓ cup
Cranberry juice	
low-cal	¾ cup
regular	¼ cup
Grapefruit juice[1]	½ cup
Grape juice	¼ cup
Nectar	⅓ cup
Orange juice[1]	½ cup

[1]–high in Vitamin C

[2]–high in Vitamin A

[3]–high in Vitamin A and Vitamin C

| Pineapple juice | ⅓ cup |
| Prune juice | ¼ cup |

Avoid

---

all sweetened frozen juice or canned fruit

Carbohydrate

Vegetables
One serving contains 25 calories
(2 grams protein, 5 grams carbohydrate)
One serving = ½ cup

Eat

Raw, baked, broiled, steamed, boiled:

Artichoke	Eggplant	String beans
Asparagus	Green pepper[3]	green or yellow
Bean sprouts	Greens, all types[3]	Summer squash[2]
Beets	Kohlrabi	Tomatoes[3]
Broccoli[3]	Mushrooms	Tomato juice[1 4]
Brussels sprouts	Okra	Turnips
Cabbage[1]	Onions	Vegetable juice
Carrots[2]	Rhubarb	cocktail[1 4]
Cauliflower[1]	Rutabaga	Water chestnuts
Celery	Sauerkraut	Zucchini[1]

Eat these raw vegetables in any quantity:

Chicory[2]	Lettuce	Radishes
Chinese cabbage	Parsley[1]	Watercress[3]
Cucumbers	Pickles[4]	Rhubarb
Endive[2]	dill or sour	
Escarole[2]		

Avoid

Creamed or fried vegetables; vegetables with gravies, sauces

[1] –high in Vitamin C
[2] –high in Vitamin A
[3] –high in Vitamin A and Vitamin C
[4] –high in salt (sodium)

Fat

Fat
One serving contains 45 calories
(5 grams of fat)

Eat

Margarine, soft tub or stick*	1 teaspoon
Margarine, diet*	3 teaspoons
Vegetable oils* (except coconut, palm)	1 teaspoon
Mayonnaise	1 teaspoon
Diet mayonnaise	3 teaspoons
Yogannaise	2 teaspoons
Avocado	⅛
Olives[4]	5
Salad dressing without sour cream or cheese (i.e., Italian, French)*-[4]	1 tablespoon
Salad dressing (low-calorie)*-[4]	2 tablespoons
Seeds (i.e., sunflower, sesame), unsalted	1 tablespoon
Nuts, unsalted	6 small
Almonds, unsalted	6
Peanuts, unsalted	10
Pecans (whole), unsalted	2

*Made with corn, cottonseed, safflower, or sunflower oil only. Choose margarine with "liquid oil" as the first listed (predominant) ingredient on the label.

Avoid

Bacon & bacon drippings[4]	Gravies, sauces, meat drippings
Butter	Hydrogenated oils (as first ingredient)
Chicken fat	
Chocolate, cocoa butter	Ice cream
Coconut & palm oil	Lard
Commercial baked goods	Margarine (regular stick)
Commercial popcorn[4] (made w/coconut oil)	Nondairy creamers w/coconut and/or palm oil

[4]–high in salt (sodium)

Creamy salad dressings[4]
(blue cheese, 1000 island,
sour cream, etc.)
Cream:
liquid, sour, whipping
(sweet)
Desserts
Dips[4] and chips[4]

Whipped topping
Nuts: cashew, macadamia
Salt pork[4]
Shortening
Sour cream
Food labeled with
nonspecific "vegetable oil"

[4]–high in salt (sodium)

Meat Tips

Ways to Trim Meat Fat

1. Eat a maximum of 8 ounces meat/fish/poultry daily. Limit beef, lamb, pork to 12 to 16 ounces per week.
2. Choose only lean cuts of meat (see list p. 99). Avoid cuts where fat is "hidden" or visible throughout the meat (i.e., brisket, rib, roast, prime rib).
3. Trim all visible fat; remove skin from poultry.
4. Bake, broil, barbecue meats; do not add fats (i.e., sauté, fry, add sauces, gravies, etc.).
5. Roast and bake meats with rack to allow excess fat to drain off meat.
6. Prepare eggs fat-free by poaching, boiling, scrambling, or cooking in nonstick pans or with nonstick sprays.
7. Remove fat from meat drippings: refrigerate drippings so that the cold fat will rise to the top and harden. Skim off or use a "gravy skimmer," which separates fat from hot drippings.
8. Weigh meat after cooking and without bone. A 3-ounce serving of cooked meat equals approximately ¼ pound (4 ounces) of raw meat.

Portions Count

3-ounce Portions

---

1 pork or veal chop, ¼" thick
2 rib lamb chops or 1 shoulder chop
leg-and-thigh or ½ breast of 3-pound chicken
1 meat pattie, 3" x ¼"
2 thin slices roast meat, each 3" x 3" x ¼"
3 medium-size pieces of stew meat
1 small beef filet or ½ small sirloin tip
1 fish filet, 3" x 3" x ½"
¼ cup tuna, salmon, crab, cottage cheese
12 medium shrimp (or 15 small)
3 boiled crabs, 15 oysters

Typical Portions

Meat, Poultry, Fish

---

3 ounces	= size of palm of lady's hand (don't count fingers!)
	= amount in a sandwich
	= amount in a "quarter pounder" (cooked)
	= chicken breast (3" across)
6 ounces	= restaurant chicken breast (6" across)
	= common luncheon or cafeteria portion
8 ounces	= common evening restaurant portion

Cheese[4]

---

1 ounce	= 1 slice on sandwich or hamburger
	= 1" cube or 1 wedge (airplane serving)
½ cup	= 1 scoop cottage cheese

---

[4]–high in salt (sodium)

A Meal Plan to Combat Hypertension

These menus have been formulated according to the following specific nutritional guidelines:

- They consist of low-sodium dishes, with approximately 2 grams (2,000 mg) of sodium per day. In every case, the diets average less than 2.3 grams of sodium per day.

- They are low-fat, with fats comprising less than 30 percent of any day's calories.

  Those foods which do contain fats have been chosen with the latest understanding of how nutrition may have an impact on hypertension. Among other things, we've emphasized the inclusion of seafoods containing polyunsaturated fish oil, a substance which may lower blood pressure.

  In this regard, a report in the April 20, 1989 issue of *The New England Journal of Medicine*, concludes that "high doses of fish oil can reduce blood pressure in men with essential hypertension. However, the clinical usefulness and safety of fish oil in the treatment of hypertension will require further study." (Knapp, Howard R., et al., "The antihypertensive effects of fish oil," Vol. 320, p. 1037).

- They are low-cholesterol, with all menus containing less than 300 mg of cholesterol per day. (In many cases, they have *far* less than 300 mg per day.)

- They are high-fiber diets, with a high percentage of daily calories (50 to 70 percent) from complex carbohydrate foods.

- They are high-calcium, typically providing from 1,000 to 1,500 mg of calcium per day.

- There is a 1,200-calorie-per-day program designed to help women lose weight. Also, a 1,500-calorie-per-day plan will enable women to maintain weight, or men to lose weight. Finally, there's a 2,200-calorie-per-day plan for men to maintain an ideal weight.

- The meals are high in potassium as a result of the high proportion of complex carbohydrates.

As I've already mentioned, these menus have been designed to be used with the food exchange system. Here is a summary of sample meal plans at three calorie levels—1,200, 1,500, 2,200—that could fit into the system. The numbers under each calorie category refer to servings from each of the exchange categories.

Food Exchanges for Sample Meal Plans

Exchanges:	1,200 cal.	1,500 cal.	2,200 cal.
Milk	1	1	2
Meat (including cheese)	5	7	8
Bread/Starch	5	7	12
Vegetables	3	3	4
Fruit	4	4	8
Fat	4	5	6

Although these exact exchanges haven't been used for every menu in this book, they should prove useful as a general guide if you plan to use the food exchange system.

Basic Tips for Using the Menus and Recipes—and for Creating Your Own Menus with the Food Exchange System

You've seen some of these tips before, as in the sections on strategies for sodium reduction. But I want to emphasize *all* the major principles at this point so that you'll be sure to have them in mind as you prepare to use the menus and recipes.

Tip 1. Be selective with protein foods, including dairy and meat products. Remember: These foods are naturally high in sodium.

For example, 1 cup of milk contains approximately 150 mg of sodium; 1 ounce of cheese has 100 to 400 mg; and 8 ounces of fresh fish, meat, or poultry have 150 mg of sodium. I suggest that you include no more than 8 ounces of meat or meat substitutes daily, and 2 to 3 low-fat milk products daily, to not consume excessive amounts of fat or cholesterol. (To check the precise nutrient content of various foods, see the charts in appendix IV.)

Tip 2. Eat large portions of fresh produce—especially fruit and vegetables. These foods contain virtually no sodium, are relatively free of fat and cholesterol, are rich in potassium and fiber, and are highly nutritious complex carbohydrates.

I recommend a minimum of six fruit and vegetable servings a day. Using the exchange system, you may want to substitute seasonal fruit in the menus.

All fresh, frozen, or canned fruits in the menus are sodium-free or low in sodium. Make it a point to buy unsalted or low-sodium canned vegetables (check the labels!).

Tip 3. Avoid canned or packaged processed foods. Most contain high levels of sodium.

Tip 4. Eat at least 4 to 6 starches daily. Most

starches—including rice, pasta, oatmeal, potatoes, and corn—are sodium-free. Prepare them without salt, even though the package instructions may recommend cooking with salt.

Tip 5. Be aware that each slice of bread contains approximately 125 mg of sodium. Instead of bread, emphasize grains such as rice, pasta, oatmeal, or oat bran. Also, it's helpful to include plenty of starches such as potatoes, corn, peas, and beans, which contain no sodium as long as they are not canned with salt. In addition, eat unsalted crackers, and avoid dry mixes for cornbread, biscuits, or muffins.

Tip 6. Do not add salt at the table—I've said this already, but I'll say it again! In cooking, use one-half as much salt as a recipe (other than those in this book) calls for, or none at all.

Tip 7. Read cereal labels. Some cereals contain approximately 300 to 600 mg of sodium per one-cup serving.

Shredded wheat, shredded wheat with extra fiber, oatmeal, cooked oat bran, puffed wheat, puffed rice, puffed corn, and special "low-sodium" labeled cereals are your best choices. Wheat-bran cereals are excellent fiber sources, but most contain high levels of sodium, so control the portion sizes of these in your diet.

Tip 8. To limit fat and cholesterol, choose fish, poultry (skinned), and meatless dishes more often (8 to 10 servings per week), and limit red-meat dishes (0 to 4 servings per week).

Tip 9. Oil and vinegar contain no sodium and often are used as salad dressing in the menus. You can purchase sodium-free bottled salad dressings in the "diet" section of most grocery stores. Or you can make your own dressings by substituting herbs and spices and sodium-free seasonings.

Tip 10. For margarine, use regular (44 mg of sodium per teaspoon), diet (22 mg sodium per teaspoon), or unsalted (no sodium), depending on your sodium restriction.

Tip 11. Choose the following as beverages: water,

mineral water, or sparkling water. Canned diet soft drinks contain a small amount of sodium—approximately 50 mg per 12-ounce can. Fruit juices are sodium-free. But V-8 and other vegetable and tomato juices are high in salt, unless you purchase the "low-sodium" varieties.

Tip 12. When cooking, avoid high-sodium condiments such as monosodium glutamate, bouillon cubes, canned broths, canned soups, meat tenderizers, garlic salt, onion salt, lemon pepper, soy sauce, teriyaki sauce, catsup, steak sauce, worcestershire sauce, and barbecue sauce.

Instead, use herbs, spices, salt-free seasoning, blends, lemon juice, tabasco sauce, Kitchen Bouquet (a liquid seasoning blend), angostura bitters, unsalted bouillon cubes, or regular wine (not cooking wine).

Note: For further information on this subject, refer to the "How to Cook with Herbs and Spices" chart on p. 234 and the "Low-Sodium Commercial Seasoning Products" on p. 242.

Tip 13. All the recipes in this book have been kitchen-tested at the Cooper Clinic. In formulating these dishes, we've substituted lower-sodium and lower-fat ingredients, including appropriate seasonings. In some cases, our nutritionists have included "*very* low sodium" recipe variations (entitled "lower sodium" variations).

Tip 14. Simply by substituting fresh goods for canned, and also herbal seasonings for salt, we've tried to avoid recipes that require special low-sodium-product purchases.

Tip 15. The use of "lite" salt in place of regular salt cuts the sodium in half. Or salt can be eliminated entirely with a "salt substitute" or "salt-free seasoning blend."

Tip 16. All recipes and menus have been computer-analyzed, using the Cooper Clinic Nutrition and Exercise Evaluation System.

Tip 17. A reminder about and expansion upon two food preparation tips that have already been suggested in other contexts:

1. Make homemade broth from defatted, unsalted chicken drippings, and freeze in ice-cube trays to be used later as "bouillon" or "broth" cubes. Regular bouillon cubes are excessive in salt.

2. In cooking, use regular wine, which is salt-free, rather than "cooking wine," which is high in sodium.

Tip 18. At salad bars, eat the fresh, simple vegetables, avoiding combination dishes (e.g., tuna salad, pasta salad, etc.). The combination plates contain unknown quantities of salt. Also avoid obvious high-salt selections such as canned bean salads, pickles, olives, croutons, bacon, commercial dressings, or salted nuts and seeds.

Tip 19. For snacks, make salt-free homemade popcorn, or purchase unsalted pretzels. Eat shredded wheat or homemade "trail mix" made of dried fruit, low-sodium cereals, and unsalted pretzels. In addition, fruit makes a good sodium-free antihypertensive snack.

Tip 20. For desserts, choose fruit, sherbet, fruit ice, frozen yogurt, ice milk, gelatin, and homemade desserts containing low-sodium ingredients. Avoid commercial pastries, cakes, and cookies, which are high in sodium.

Tip 21. Avoid fast foods or follow the fast food guidelines on p. 92. Choose mainly salad bars and baked potatoes. Top potatoes with vegetables from the salad bar, including green pepper, onions, mushrooms, and broccoli.

Tip 22. Prepare sandwiches with leftover unsalted chicken, meat, or other such foods. Avoid cured, processed luncheon meats. For example: 3 ounces of chicken contain 75 mg of sodium, while 3 ounces of salami or ham have 1,200 mg of sodium!

Go easy on or omit mayonnaise and mustard: They tend to be high in sodium. Skip the pickles and olives, and use unsalted pretzels instead of chips. Fresh fruit and raw carrot sticks are also a good antihypertensive way to fill out a sandwich meal.

Tip 23. For adequate calcium, include 2 to 3 nonfat or low-fat milk products daily (e.g., milk, yogurt, or cheese). Part-skim-milk mozzarella is an excellent lower-sodium, low-fat, high-calcium cheese. Deli cheese counters may include many specialty low-fat, low-sodium cheeses—but read the labels to find out which ones are best.

Finally, be aware that low-fat cottage cheese is high in sodium, though it is a good source of calcium.

Tip 24. In the menus, "diet" margarine or mayonnaise

refers to products labeled "low-calorie" or "50 calories per tablespoon." Tub, unsalted diet margarine is the best choice for a low-sodium, low-fat, low-calorie meal plan.

Tip 25. Prepare homemade beans from scratch. If you must use canned beans occasionally, rinse them first to reduce their sodium content.

Daily Menus
The Antihypertensive
Meal Plan

1,200 - Calorie Menus

Week 1—Monday

Breakfast

1 cup cooked oat bran cereal without salt (2 Bread)
2 tablespoons raisins (1 Fruit)
1 cup skim milk (1 Milk)

Lunch

1 pita pocket sandwich:
　　1 whole wheat pita pocket (2 Bread)
　　1 ounce sliced turkey (1 Meat)
　　½ ounce part-skim mozzarella cheese (½ Meat)
　　1 teaspoon mayonnaise (1 Fat)
　　½ teaspoon mustard
　　shredded lettuce and ½ cup chopped tomatoes (1
　　　　Vegetable)
1 small apple (1 Fruit)
½ cup skim milk (½ Milk)

Dinner

¾ cup Gazpacho (1½ Vegetable, ½ Fat)(24 mg Sodium), see p. 157,
¼ sliced avocado (2 Fat)
1 Pita Cracker (⅛ Bread) (23 mg Sodium), see p. 338
1 cup Spanish Chicken and Rice (3½ Meat, 2 Bread, 1 Fat, 2 Vegetable) (375 mg Sodium), see p. 166
12 large green grapes (1 Fruit)

Week 1—Tuesday

Breakfast

½ cup fresh orange slices (1 Fruit)
1 poached egg (1 Meat)
1 slice whole wheat toast (1 Bread)
1 teaspoon unsalted margarine (1 Fat)
1 tablespoon apple butter (½ Fruit)
1 cup skim milk (1 Milk)

Lunch

1 cup Cold Pasta Salad (1½ Bread, ½ Meat, 2 Vegetable, ½ Fat) (412 mg Sodium), see p. 160
1 slice garlic bread:
   1 3-inch slice Italian bread (1 Bread)
   1 teaspoon unsalted margarine (1 Fat)
   ½ teaspoon garlic powder
1 sliced kiwi (2 Fruit)

Dinner

2½ ounces Peppered Veal (2½ Meat, 1 Vegetable, ½ Bread, ½ Fat) (208 mg Sodium), see p. 167
1 small baked potato (1 Bread) with
1 teaspoon unsalted margarine (1 Fat)
½ cup steamed broccoli (1 Vegetable) seasoned with
1 teaspoon pimiento
½ cup unsweetened applesauce (1 Fruit)

Week 1—Wednesday

Breakfast

½ cup unsweetened orange juice (1 Fruit)
½ cup bran flakes (1 Bread)
1 cup skim milk (1 Milk)
½ cup unsweetened, canned peaches (1 Fruit)

Lunch

1 grilled cheese sandwich:
 2 slices whole wheat bread (2 Bread)
 1½ ounces low-fat cheese (1½ Meat), grilled using
 2 teaspoons unsalted margarine (2 Fat)
 3 slices tomato (1 Vegetable)
1½ cups fresh strawberries (2 Fruit)
½ cup skim milk (½ Milk)

Dinner

3 ounces Herbed Garlic Fish Fillets (3 Meat) (202 mg
 Sodium), see p. 169
½ cup Oven French Fries (2 Bread) (5 mg Sodium), see
 p. 183
1 orange romaine salad:
 2 cups romaine lettuce (2 Vegetable)
 ½ cup unsweetened mandarin oranges (1 Fruit)
 1 teaspoon rice vinegar
 1 teaspoon olive oil (1 Fat)
1 whole wheat dinner roll (1 Bread)
½ cup skim milk (½ Milk)

Week 1—Thursday

Breakfast

1 cup unsweetened, canned pears (2 Fruit)
1 vegetable omelet:
 1 egg (1 Meat)
 1 slice tomato
 2 fresh sliced mushrooms
 1 chopped green onion (tomato, mushrooms, onion =
  1 Vegetable)
1 whole wheat English muffin (2 Bread)
2 teaspoons unsalted margarine (2 Fat)
½ cup skim milk (½ Milk)

Lunch

1 "Munchie Tray":
    1 ounce sliced chicken (1 Meat)
    ½ ounce low-fat cheese (½ Meat)
    12 saltine crackers, unsalted tops (2 Bread)
    12 large green grapes (1 Fruit)
1 cup Fruit Smoothy (1½ Milk) (85 mg Sodium), see p. 181

Dinner

1 Spicy Bean Enchilada (1 Meat, 2 Bread, ½ Vegetable) (553 mg Sodium), see p. 176
1 cup tossed dinner salad (1 Vegetable)
1½ tablespoons oil and vinegar dressing (1½ Fat)

Week 1—Friday

Breakfast

1 cup cooked oatmeal or oat bran cereal without salt (2 Bread)
½ mashed banana (1 Fruit)
1 cup skim milk (1 Milk)

Lunch

½ cup Long Grain and Wild Rice Chicken Salad (1 Meat, 1 Bread, ½ Vegetable, ½ Fruit, 1 Fat) (250 mg Sodium), see p. 161, on
¼ cup shredded lettuce
6 saltine crackers, unsalted tops (1 Bread)

Dinner

1 piece Vegetarian Lasagna (2 Bread, 2 Meat, 2½ Vegetable, ½ Fat) (350 mg Sodium), see p. 179
1 whole wheat dinner roll (1 Bread)
2 teaspoons unsalted margarine (2 Fat)
½ cup fresh fruit salad (1 Fruit)
½ cup skim milk (½ Milk)

Week 1—Saturday

Breakfast

1 slice French Toast Puff
(1 Meat, ⅛ Milk, ½ Fruit, 1 Bread) (230 mg Sodium), see p. 154, with
1 teaspoon unsalted margarine (1 Fat) and
2 tablespoons Berry Syrup (1 Fruit) (0 mg Sodium), see p. 185
1 cup skim milk (1 Milk)

Lunch

½ cup Tuna Salad (2 Meat, 1 Milk) (707 mg Sodium), see p. 162, on
1 lettuce leaf with 3 slices tomato (1 Vegetable)
4 pieces melba toast (1 Bread)
1 medium apple (2 Fruit)
½ cup skim milk (½ Milk)

Dinner

3 Stuffed Shells (1 Meat, 2 Bread, 3 Vegetable, ½ Fat) (150 mg Sodium), see p. 178
1 cup tossed dinner salad with cucumber and carrot slices (1 Vegetable)
1 tablespoon oil and vinegar dressing (1 Fat)

Week 1—Sunday

Breakfast

1 Oatmeal Pancake (1 Bread, 1/6 Milk) (199 mg Sodium), see p. 156
1 teaspoon unsalted margarine (1 Fat)
1 tablespoon low-calorie syrup (¼ Fruit)
1 cup skim milk (1 Milk)

Lunch

1 fruit salad:
   ¾ cup fresh strawberries (1 Fruit)
   12 large green grapes (1 Fruit)
   1 sliced banana (2 Fruit)
¼ cup low-fat cottage cheese (1 Meat)
6 saltine crackers, unsalted tops (1 Bread)

Dinner

4 ounces Teriyaki Steak (4 Meat, ½ Vegetable, ½ Fat)
   (472 mg Sodium), see p. 174
¾ cup steamed rice (1½ Bread) with
1 teaspoon unsalted margarine (1 Fat)
1 cup stir-fry vegetables:
   ¼ cup julienne zucchini (½ Vegetable)
   ¼ cup julienne carrots (½ Vegetable)
   ¼ cup chopped red bell peppers (½ Vegetable)
   ¼ cup sliced onion (½ Vegetable)
   1 teaspoon safflower oil (1 Fat)
   ¼ teaspoon ginger powder
   ¼ teaspoon minced garlic
½ cup skim milk (½ Milk)

Week 2—Monday

Breakfast

1 waffle (1 Bread, 1 Fat) topped with
½ cup unsweetened applesauce (1 Fruit) and
½ teaspoon cinnamon
1 cup skim milk (1 Milk)

Lunch

1 small baked potato (1 Bread) topped with
2 tablespoons grated cheddar cheese (½ Meat)
1 cup fresh fruit salad (2 Fruit)

Dinner

3 ounces Grilled Sesame Chicken Breast (3 Meat, ½ Fat, ½ Fruit) (443 mg Sodium), see p. 164
½ cup cooked corkscrew pasta (1 Bread) with
1 teaspoon unsalted margarine (1 Fat)
½ cup steamed broccoli (1 Vegetable)
1 cup marinated vegetables:
  ½ cup sliced tomato
  ½ cup sliced cucumber (tomato and cucumber = 1 Vegetable)
  1 tablespoon Italian dressing (1 Fat)

Week 2—Tuesday

Breakfast

½ cup unsweetened orange juice (1 Fruit)
1 Oat Bran Muffin (½ Bread, ½ Fruit, ½ Fat) (60 mg Sodium), see p. 155
¼ cup scrambled egg substitute (1 Meat) cooked with vegetable oil cooking spray
1 teaspoon unsalted margarine (1 Fat)

Lunch

1 cup Low-Sodium Minestrone Soup (1 Bread, 1 Vegetable) (57 mg Sodium), see p. 157
1 turkey sandwich:
  2 slices diet whole wheat bread (1 Bread)
  1 ounce sliced turkey breast (1 Meat)
  1 teaspoon diet mayonnaise (½ Fat)
  ¼ cup alfalfa sprouts (1 Vegetable)
1 cup plain, nonfat yogurt (1 Milk) with
1 teaspoon sugar substitute and
1 teaspoon vanilla
¾ cup fresh strawberries (1 Fruit)

Dinner

1¾ cups Low-Sodium Shrimp Creole (2 Meat, 1½
    Bread, 2 Vegetable) (291 mg Sodium), see p. 171
1 3-inch slice French bread (1 Bread)
1 teaspoon unsalted margarine (1 Fat)
Lettuce wedge with
1 tablespoon French dressing (1 Fat)
1 small baked apple (1 Fruit)

Week 2—Wednesday

Breakfast

1 English muffin (2 Bread)
3 teaspoons unsalted diet margarine (1 Fat)
1 fresh fruit cup:
    ¼ sliced banana (½ Fruit)
    ½ sliced orange (½ Fruit)
1 cup homemade cocoa:
    1 cup heated skim milk (1 Milk)
    1 tablespoon cocoa
    1 teaspoon sugar substitute

Lunch

1 tostada:
    1 flour tortilla (1 Bread)
    ¼ cup cooked, drained ground beef (1 Meat)
    1 tablespoon picante sauce
    2 tablespoons grated cheddar cheese (½ Meat)
    ¼ cup chopped tomato (½ Vegetable)
½ cantaloupe (2 Fruit)

Dinner

2 ounces Veal Scaloppine (2 Meat, 1 Vegetable, 1 Fat, 1 Bread) (168 mg Sodium), see p. 168
½ cup cooked egg noodles (1 Bread)
½ cup steamed green beans (1 Vegetable)
1 cup romaine lettuce with
1 tablespoon oil and vinegar dressing (1 Fat)
½ cup unsweetened, canned pears (1 Fruit)

Week 2—Thursday

Breakfast

1 Bran Muffin (1 Bread, ½ Fruit, 1 Fat) (200 mg Sodium), see p. 153
¼ cup scrambled egg substitute (1 Meat) cooked with vegetable oil cooking spray
½ fresh grapefruit (1 Fruit)

Lunch

½ cup cooked spaghetti (1 Bread)
½ cup Low-Sodium Italian Tomato Sauce (1½ Vegetable) (20 mg Sodium), see p. 185
1½ tablespoons grated Parmesan cheese (½ Meat)
1 small fresh peach (1 Fruit)

Dinner

¾ serving Low-Sodium Beef Broccoli Stir-Fry (3 Meat, 1 Vegetable) (408 mg Sodium), see p. 172
½ cup cooked rice (1 Bread)
1 oriental salad:
  1 cup mixed greens
  ½ cup unsweetened mandarin oranges (1 Fruit)
  1 tablespoon slivered almonds (1 Fat)
  2 teaspoons oil and vinegar dressing (1 Fat)
1 cup Apple Oat Crisp (2 Fruit, 1 Bread, ½ Fat) (80 mg Sodium), see p. 180

Week 2–Friday

Breakfast

½ cup unsweetened grapefruit juice (1 Fruit)
¾ cup corn bran cereal (1 Bread)
1 cup skim milk (1 Milk)
1 slice whole wheat toast (1 Bread)
1 teaspoon unsalted margarine (1 Fat)

Lunch

1 serving Low-Sodium Seafood Quiche (½ Milk, 2½
    Meat) (350 mg Sodium), see p. 170
½ cup steamed asparagus (1 Vegetable)
½ cup Apple Waldorf Salad (1 Fruit, 1 Fat) (76 mg So-
    dium), see p. 159
1 whole wheat dinner roll (1 Bread)
1 teaspoon unsalted margarine (1 Fat)

Dinner

2 tacos:
    2 taco shells (1 Bread, 1 Fat)
    ½ cup cooked, seasoned ground chicken (2 Meat)
    ¼ cup chopped tomato (½ Vegetable)
    shredded lettuce
    picante sauce
½ cup steamed zucchini (1 Vegetable)
½ cup sugar-free vanilla pudding (½ Milk) with
½ sliced banana (1 Fruit) and
4 vanilla wafers (1 Bread)

Week 2—Saturday

Breakfast

½ cup unsweetened orange juice (1 Fruit)
½ cup cooked oatmeal without salt (1 Bread)
1 cup skim milk (1 Milk)

Lunch

1 serving Ricotta-Parmesan Torte (1 Fat, ½ Vegetable,
    1½ Bread, 1 Meat) (365 mg Sodium), see p. 175
1 cup steamed, mixed vegetables (2 Vegetable)
1 teaspoon unsalted margarine (1 Fat)
12 large green grapes (1 Fruit)
1 cup skim milk (1 Milk)

Dinner

4 ounces Low-Sodium Southern Fried Chicken (4 Meat,
    ½ Bread, ½ Fat) (98 mg Sodium), see p. 165
½ cup mashed potatoes (1 Bread)
½ cup steamed French-cut green beans (1 Vegetable)
½ cup fresh pineapple (1 Fruit)
1 teaspoon unsalted margarine (1 Fat)

Week 2—Sunday

Breakfast

½ cup unsweetened grapefruit juice (1 Fruit)
½ English muffin (1 Bread) topped with
½ small sliced apple (½ Fruit) and
2 tablespoons grated cheddar cheese (½ Meat)
¾ cup bran flakes (1 Bread)
1 cup skim milk (1 Milk)

Lunch

1 chicken salad sandwich:
    2 slices diet whole wheat bread (1 Bread)
    ¼ cup cooked, chopped chicken (1 Meat)
    2 tablespoons diet mayonnaise (2 Fat)
6 raw carrot sticks (1 Vegetable)
1 small fresh pear (1 Fruit)
¾ cup skim milk (¾ Milk)

Dinner

2 ounces Shishkabob (2 Meat, 1 Vegetable) (196 mg
    Sodium), see p. 173
1 small baked potato (1 Bread) with
1 tablespoon sour cream (1 Fat) and
1 teaspoon chives
½ cup steamed broccoli (1 Vegetable)
¼ honeydew melon (2 Fruit)

1,500 - Calorie Menus

Week 1—Monday

Breakfast

1 cup cooked oat bran cereal without salt (2 Bread)
2 tablespoons raisins (1 Fruit)
½ cup skim milk (½ Milk)

Lunch

1 pita pocket sandwich:
    1 whole wheat pita pocket (2 Bread)
    1 ounce sliced turkey (1 Meat)
    ½ ounce part-skim mozzarella cheese (½ Meat)
    1 teaspoon mayonnaise (1 Fat)
    ½ teaspoon mustard
    shredded lettuce and ½ cup chopped tomatoes (1
        Vegetable)
1 large apple (3 Fruit)

Dinner

¾ cup Gazpacho (1½ Vegetable, ½ Fat) (24 mg So-
    dium), see p. 157, with
¼ sliced avocado (2 Fat)
1 Pita Cracker (⅛ Bread) (23 mg Sodium), see p. 338
1 cup Spanish Chicken and Rice (3½ Meat, 2 Bread, 2
    Vegetable, 1 Fat), (375 mg Sodium), see p. 166
24 large green grapes (2 Fruit)

Snack

1 cup plain, nonfat yogurt (1 Milk)
½ cup unsweetened, crushed pineapple (1 Fruit)
2 vanilla wafers (½ Bread)

Week 1—Tuesday

Breakfast

½ cup fresh orange slices (1 Fruit)
1 poached egg (1 Meat)
1 slice whole wheat toast (1 Bread)
1 teaspoon unsalted margarine (1 Fat)
1 tablespoon apple butter (½ Fruit)
1 cup skim milk (1 Milk)

Lunch

1½ cups Cold Pasta Salad (2¼ Bread, ¾ Meat, 3 Vegetable, ¾ Fat) (618 mg Sodium), see p. 160
2 slices garlic bread:
   2 3-inch slices Italian bread (1 Bread)
   1 teaspoon unsalted margarine (1 Fat)
   ½ teaspoon garlic powder
1 sliced kiwi (2 Fruit)

Dinner

2½ ounces Peppered Veal (2½ Meat, 1 Vegetable, ½ Bread, ½ Fat) (208 mg Sodium), see p. 168
1 small baked potato (1 Bread) with
1 teaspoon unsalted margarine (1 Fat) and
¼ cup plain, nonfat yogurt (¼ Milk)
½ cup steamed broccoli (1 Vegetable) seasoned with
1 teaspoon pimiento
½ cup unsweetened applesauce (1 Fruit)

Week 1—Wednesday

Breakfast

½ cup unsweetened orange juice (1 Fruit)
½ cup shredded wheat biscuits (1 Bread)
1 cup skim milk (1 Milk)
1 cup unsweetened, canned peaches (2 Fruit)

Lunch

1 grilled cheese sandwich:
  2 slices whole wheat bread (2 Bread)
  2 ounces low-fat cheese (2 Meat), grilled using
  2 teaspoons unsalted margarine (2 Fat)
  3 slices tomato (1 Vegetable)
1½ cups fresh strawberries (2 Fruit)
½ cup skim milk (½ Milk)

Dinner

3 ounces Herbed Garlic Fish Fillets (3 Meat) (202 mg
    Sodium), see p. 169
1 cup Oven French Fries (4 Bread) (10 mg Sodium),
    see p. 183
1 orange romaine salad:
  2 cups romaine lettuce (2 Vegetable)
  ½ cup unsweetened mandarin oranges (1 Fruit)
  1 teaspoon rice vinegar
  1 teaspoon olive oil (1 Fat)
1 whole wheat dinner roll (1 Bread)
1 teaspoon unsalted margarine (1 Fat)

Snack

½ cup ice milk (1 Milk)

Week 1—Thursday

Breakfast

1 cup unsweetened, canned pears (2 Fruit)
1 vegetable omelet:
    1 whole egg, plus 2 egg whites (2 Meat)
    3 slices tomato
    2 fresh sliced mushrooms
    1 chopped green onion
    (tomato, mushrooms, onion = 1½ Vegetable)
1 whole wheat English muffin (2 Bread)
2 teaspoons unsalted margarine (2 Fat)

Lunch

1 "Munchie Tray":
    1 ounce sliced chicken (1 Meat)
    ½ ounce low-fat cheese (½ Meat)
    9 saltine crackers, unsalted tops (1½ Bread)
    12 large green grapes (1 Fruit)
1 cup Fruit Smoothy (1½ Milk) (85 mg Sodium), see p. 181

Dinner

1 Spicy Bean Enchilada (1 Meat, 2 Bread, ½ Vegetable) (553 mg Sodium), see p. 176
1 cup steamed rice (2 Bread) mixed with
¼ cup tomato sauce (1 Vegetable)
1 cup tossed dinner salad (1 Vegetable)
2 tablespoons oil and vinegar dressing (2 Fat)

Snack

1 large orange (2 Fruit)

Week 1—Friday

Breakfast

1 cup cooked oatmeal or oat bran cereal without salt (2
    Bread)
½ mashed banana (1 Fruit)
1 cup skim milk (1 Milk)

Lunch

1 cup Long Grain and Wild Rice Chicken Salad (2 Meat,
    2 Bread, 1 Vegetable, 1 Fruit, 2 Fat) (500 mg So-
    dium), see p. 161 on
¼ cup shredded lettuce
6 saltine crackers, unsalted tops (1 Bread)

Dinner

1 piece Vegetarian Lasagna (2 Bread, 2 Meat, 2½ Vege-
    table, ½ Fat) (350 mg Sodium), see p. 179
1 whole wheat dinner roll (1 Bread)
2 teaspoons unsalted margarine (2 Fat)
1 cup fresh fruit salad (2 Fruit)
1 cup skim milk (1 Milk)

Week 1—Saturday

Breakfast

½ cup orange juice (1 Fruit)
1 slice French Toast Puff
        (1 Meat, ⅛ Milk, ½ Fruit, 1 Bread) (230 mg So-
        dium), see p. 154, with
1 teaspoon unsalted margarine (1 Fat) and
½ cup plain, nonfat yogurt (½ Milk) and
4 tablespoons Berry Syrup (2 Fruit) (0 mg Sodium), see
    p. 185
½ cup skim milk (½ Milk)

Lunch

½ cup Tuna Salad (2 Meat, 1 Milk) (707 mg Sodium),
    see p. 162, on
1 lettuce leaf with 3 slices tomato (1 Vegetable)
4 pieces melba toast (1 Bread)
1 large apple (3 Fruit)
½ cup skim milk (½ Milk)

Dinner

3 Stuffed Shells (1 Meat, 2 Bread, 3 Vegetable, ½ Fat)
    (150 mg Sodium), see p. 178
½ cup steamed broccoli (1 Vegetable) with
1 teaspoon unsalted margarine (1 Fat)
1 cup tossed dinner salad with cucumber and carrot
    slices (1 Vegetable)
1 tablespoon oil and vinegar dressing (1 Fat)

Snack

1 small oatmeal cookie (1 Bread)

Week 1—Sunday

Breakfast

2 Oatmeal Pancakes (2 Bread, ⅓ Milk) (398 mg So-
    dium), see p. 156
1 teaspoon unsalted margarine (1 Fat)
2 tablespoons low-calorie syrup (½ Fruit)
1 cup skim milk (1 Milk)

Lunch

1 fruit salad:
    ¾ cup fresh strawberries (1 Fruit)
    12 large green grapes (1 Fruit)
    1 sliced banana (2 Fruit)
    1 small sliced apple (1 Fruit)
½ cup low-fat cottage cheese (2 Meat)
6 saltine crackers, unsalted tops (1 Bread)

Dinner

4 ounces Teriyaki Steak (4 Meat, ½ Vegetable, ½ Fat)
    (472 mg Sodium), see p. 174
1 cup steamed rice (2 Bread) with
1 teaspoon unsalted margarine (1 Fat)
1 cup stir-fry vegetables:
    ¼ cup julienne zucchini (½ Vegetable)
    ¼ cup julienne carrots (½ Vegetable)
    ¼ cup chopped red bell peppers (½ Vegetable)
    ¼ cup sliced onion (½ Vegetable)
    1 teaspoon safflower oil (1 Fat)
    ¼ teaspoon ginger powder
    ¼ teaspoon minced garlic
1 cup skim milk (1 Milk)

Snack

½ cup unsalted pretzel sticks (1 Bread)

Week 2—Monday

Breakfast

¾ cup unsweetened orange-grapefruit juice (1½ Fruit)
1 waffle (1 Bread, 1 Fat) topped with
½ cup unsweetened applesauce (1 Fruit) and
1 teaspoon cinnamon
1 cup skim milk (1 Milk)

Lunch

1 small baked potato (1 Bread) topped with
2 tablespoons grated cheddar cheese (½ Meat)
1 cup fresh fruit salad (2 Fruit) with
¼ cup low-fat cottage cheese (1 Meat)

Dinner

3 ounces Grilled Sesame Chicken Breast (3 Meat, ½ Fat, ½ Fruit) (443 mg Sodium), see p. 164
1 cup cooked corkscrew pasta (2 Bread) with
1 teaspoon unsalted margarine (1 Fat)
½ cup steamed broccoli (1 Vegetable)
1 cup marinated vegetables:
  ½ cup sliced tomato
  ½ cup sliced cucumber
  (tomato and cucumber = 1 Vegetable)
  1 tablespoon Italian dressing (1 Fat)
¼ cantaloupe (1 Fruit)

Week 2—Tuesday

Breakfast

½ cup unsweetened orange juice (1 Fruit)
1 Oat Bran Muffin (½ Bread, ½ Fruit, ½ Fat) (60 mg Sodium), see p. 155
¼ cup scrambled egg substitute (1 Meat) cooked with vegetable oil cooking spray
1 teaspoon unsalted margarine (1 Fat)
1 cup skim milk (1 Milk)

Lunch

1 cup Low-Sodium Minestrone Soup (1 Bread, 1 Vegetable) (57 mg Sodium), see p. 157
1 turkey sandwich:
  2 slices whole wheat bread (2 Bread)
  2 ounces sliced turkey breast (2 Meat)
  1 teaspoon diet mayonnaise (½ Fat)
  ¼ cup alfalfa sprouts (1 Vegetable)
  1 slice tomato (½ Vegetable)
1 cup plain, nonfat yogurt (1 Milk) with
1 teaspoon sugar substitute and
1 teaspoon vanilla
¾ cup fresh strawberries (1 Fruit)

Dinner

2½ cups Low-Sodium Shrimp Creole (3 Meat, 2 Bread,
    3 Vegetable) (436 mg Sodium), see p. 171
1 3-inch slice French bread (1 Bread)
1 teaspoon unsalted margarine (1 Fat)
Lettuce wedge with
1 tablespoon French dressing (1 Fat)
1 small baked apple (1 Fruit)

Week 2—Wednesday

Breakfast

1 English muffin (2 Bread)
3 teaspoons unsalted diet margarine (1 Fat)
1 fresh fruit cup:
    ¼ sliced banana (½ Fruit)
    ½ sliced orange (½ Fruit)
1 cup homemade cocoa:
    1 cup heated skim milk (1 Milk)
    1 tablespoon cocoa
    1 teaspoon sugar substitute

Lunch

2 tostadas:
    2 flour tortillas (2 Bread)
    ¼ cup cooked, drained ground beef (1 Meat)
    2 tablespoons picante sauce
    2 tablespoons grated cheddar cheese (½ Meat)
    ½ cup chopped tomato (1 Vegetable)
¼ cantaloupe (1 Fruit)

Dinner

3 ounces Veal Scaloppine (3 Meat, 1½ Vegetable, 1 Fat,
    1 Bread) (252 mg Sodium), see p. 168
½ cup cooked egg noodles (1 Bread)
½ cup steamed green beans (1 Vegetable)
1 cup romaine lettuce with
1 tablespoon oil and vinegar dressing (1 Fat)
½ cup unsweetened, canned pears (1 Fruit)
1 cup skim milk (1 Milk)

Week 2—Thursday

Breakfast

1 Bran Muffin (1 Bread, ½ Fruit, 1 Fat) (200 mg So-
    dium), see p. 155
1 teaspoon unsalted margarine (1 Fat)
¼ cup scrambled egg substitute (1 Meat) cooked with
    vegetable oil cooking spray
½ fresh grapefruit (1 Fruit)
1 cup skim milk (1 Milk)

Lunch

¾ cup cooked spaghetti (1½ Bread)
½ cup Low-Sodium Italian Tomato Sauce (1½ Vegeta-
    ble) (20 mg Sodium), see p. 185
1½ tablespoons grated Parmesan cheese (½ Meat)
1 3-inch slice French bread (1 Bread)
1 small fresh peach (1 Fruit)
1 cup skim milk (1 Milk)

Dinner

1 serving Low-Sodium Beef Broccoli Stir-Fry (4 Meat, 2
    Vegetable, ½ Fat) (544 mg Sodium), see p. 172
½ cup cooked rice (1 Bread)
1 oriental salad:
    1 cup mixed greens
    ½ cup unsweetened mandarin oranges (1 Fruit)
    1 tablespoon slivered almonds (1 Fat)
    1 tablespoon oil and vinegar dressing (1 Fat)
1 cup Apple Oat Crisp (2 Fruit, 1 Bread, ½ Fat) (80 mg
    Sodium), see p. 180

Week 2—Friday

Breakfast

½ cup unsweetened grapefruit juice (1 Fruit)
¾ cup corn bran cereal (1 Bread)
½ cup fresh blueberries (1 Fruit)
1 cup skim milk (1 Milk)
1 slice whole wheat toast (1 Bread)
1 teaspoon unsalted margarine (1 Fat)

Lunch

1 serving Low-Sodium Seafood Quiche (½ Milk, 2½
    Meat) (350 mg Sodium), see p. 170
½ cup steamed asparagus (1 Vegetable)
½ cup Apple Waldorf Salad (1 Fruit, 1 Fat) (76 mg So-
    dium), see p. 159
2 whole wheat dinner rolls (2 Bread)
1 teaspoon unsalted margarine (1 Fat)

Dinner

2 tacos:
    2 taco shells (1 Bread, 1 Fat)
    ½ cup cooked, seasoned ground chicken (2 Meat)
    ¼ cup chopped tomato (½ Vegetable)
    shredded lettuce
    picante sauce
½ cup steamed zucchini (1 Vegetable)
½ cup sugar-free vanilla pudding (½ Milk) with
½ sliced banana (1 Fruit) and
4 vanilla wafers (1 Bread)

Week 2—Saturday

Breakfast

½ cup unsweetened orange juice (1 Fruit)
½ cup cooked oatmeal without salt (1 Bread)
1 slice whole wheat toast (1 Bread)
3 teaspoons unsalted diet margarine (1 Fat)
1 cup skim milk (1 Milk)

Lunch

1 serving Ricotta-Parmesan Torte (1 Fat, ½ Vegetable,
    1½ Bread, 1 Meat) (365 mg Sodium), see p. 175
2 4-inch breadsticks (1 Bread)
1 cup steamed, mixed vegetables (2 Vegetable)
1 teaspoon unsalted margarine (1 Fat)
½ cup Turkey-Fruit Salad (1 Meat, 1 Fruit, ½ Vegeta-
    ble) (75 mg Sodium), see p. 163
6 large green grapes (½ Fruit)
1 cup skim milk (1 Milk)

Dinner

3 ounces Low-Sodium Southern Fried Chicken (3 Meat,
  ½ Bread, ½ Fat) (195 mg Sodium), see p. 165
½ cup mashed potatoes (1 Bread)
½ cup steamed French-cut green beans (1 Vegetable)
1 cup fresh pineapple (2 Fruit)
1 teaspoon unsalted margarine (1 Fat)

Week 2—Sunday

Breakfast

½ cup unsweetened grapefruit juice (1 Fruit)
1 English muffin (2 Bread) topped with
1 small sliced apple (1 Fruit) and
1 tablespoon grated cheddar cheese (¼ Meat)
¾ cup bran flakes (1 Bread)
1 cup skim milk (1 Milk)

Lunch

1 chicken salad sandwich:
  2 slices whole wheat bread (2 Bread)
  ¼ cup cooked, chopped chicken (1 Meat)
  2 tablespoons diet mayonnaise (2 Fat)
6 raw carrot sticks (1 Vegetable)
1 small fresh pear (1 Fruit)
1 cup skim milk (1 Milk)

Dinner

3 ounces Shishkabob (3 Meat, 2 Vegetable) (295 mg
  Sodium), see p. 173
1 small baked potato (1 Bread) with
1 tablespoon sour cream (1 Fat) and
1 teaspoon chives
½ cup steamed broccoli (1 Vegetable)
¼ honeydew melon (2 Fruit)

2,200 - Calorie Menus

Week 1—Monday

Breakfast

1 cup orange juice (2 Fruit)
1 cup cooked oat bran cereal without salt (2 Bread)
2 tablespoons raisins (1 Fruit)
1 cup skim milk (1 Milk)

Lunch

1 pita pocket sandwich:
  1 whole wheat pita pocket (2 Bread)
  1 ounce sliced turkey (1 Meat)
  ½ ounce part-skim mozzarella cheese (½ Meat)
  2 teaspoons mayonnaise (2 Fat)
  ½ teaspoon mustard
  shredded lettuce and
    ½ cup chopped tomatoes (1 Vegetable)
1 large apple (3 Fruit)
½ cup skim milk (½ Milk)

Dinner

1½ cups Gazpacho (3 Vegetable, 1 Fat) (48 mg Sodium), see p. 157 with
¼ sliced avocado (2 Fat)
4 Pita Crackers (½ Bread) (92 mg Sodium), see p. 338
1½ cups Spanish Chicken and Rice (5¼ Meat, 3 Bread, 3 Vegetable, 1½ Fat), (563 mg Sodium), see p. 166
24 large green grapes (2 Fruit)

Snack

1 cup plain, nonfat yogurt
    (1 Milk)
½ cup unsweetened, crushed pineapple (1 Fruit)
4 vanilla wafers (1 Bread)

Week 1—Tuesday

Breakfast

1 cup fresh orange slices (2 Fruit)
¼ cup scrambled egg substitute (1 Meat) cooked with
    vegetable oil cooking spray
2 slices whole wheat toast (2 Bread)
1 teaspoon unsalted margarine (1 Fat)
1 tablespoon apple butter (½ Fruit)
1 cup skim milk (1 Milk)

Lunch

2 cups Cold Pasta Salad (3 Bread, 1 Meat, 4 Vegetable,
    1 Fat) (824 mg Sodium), see p. 160
2 slices garlic bread:
    2 3-inch slices Italian bread (2 Bread)
    2 teaspoons unsalted margarine (2 Fat)
    ½ teaspoon garlic powder
1 sliced kiwi (2 Fruit)

Dinner

5 ounces Peppered Veal (5 Meat, 2 Vegetable, 1 Bread,
    1 Fat) (416 mg Sodium), see p. 167
1 small baked potato (1 Bread) with
1 teaspoon unsalted margarine (1 Fat) and
¼ cup plain, nonfat yogurt (¼ Milk)
½ cup steamed broccoli (1 Vegetable)
½ cup unsweetened applesauce (1 Fruit)

Snack

½ cup plain, nonfat yogurt (½ Milk) with
½ cup fresh blueberries (1 Fruit)

Week 1—Wednesday

Breakfast

1 cup unsweetened orange juice (2 Fruit)
½ cup shredded wheat biscuits (1 Bread)
1 cup skim milk (1 Milk)
1 cup unsweetened, canned peaches (2 Fruit)

Lunch

1 grilled tuna melt:
    2 slices whole wheat bread (2 Bread)
    ½ cup tuna, packed in water, low-sodium (2 Meat)
      mixed with
    2 teaspoons mayonnaise (2 Fat)
    2 ounces American cheese (2 Meat), grilled using
    1 teaspoon unsalted margarine (1 Fat)
3 slices tomato (1 Vegetable)
1 cup raw broccoli and cauliflower (1 Vegetable)
1½ cups fresh strawberries (2 Fruit)
½ cup skim milk (½ Milk)

Dinner

6 ounces Herbed Garlic Fish Fillets (6 Meat) (404 mg
    Sodium), see p. 169
1 cup Oven French Fries (4 Bread) (10 mg Sodium),
    see p. 337
1 orange romaine salad:
    2 cups romaine lettuce (2 Vegetable)
    1 cup unsweetened mandarin oranges (2 Fruit)
    1 teaspoon rice vinegar
    1 teaspoon olive oil (1 Fat)
1 whole wheat dinner roll (1 Bread)
1 teaspoon unsalted margarine (1 Fat)

Snack

½ cup ice milk (1 Milk)
½ cup fresh raspberries (1 Fruit)
25 small unsalted pretzel sticks (1 Bread)

Week 1—Thursday

Breakfast

1 cup unsweetened, canned pears (2 Fruit)
1 vegetable omelet:
    ¾ cup egg substitute (3 Meat)
    3 slices tomato
    2 fresh sliced mushrooms
    1 chopped green onion
    (tomato, mushrooms, onion = 1½ Vegetable)
    ¼ teaspoon dried oregano
1 whole wheat English muffin (2 Bread)
2 teaspoons unsalted margarine (2 Fat)

Lunch

1 "Munchie Tray":
    4 ounces sliced chicken (4 Meat)
    12 saltine crackers, unsalted tops (2 Bread)
    24 large green grapes (2 Fruit)
    ½ cup raw carrot sticks (½ Vegetable)
    ½ cup raw celery sticks (½ Vegetable)
1 cup Fruit Smoothy (1½ Milk) (85 mg Sodium), see p. 181

Dinner

1 Spicy Bean Enchilada (1 Meat, 2 Bread, ½ Vegetable) (553 mg Sodium), see p. 176
1½ cups steamed rice (3 Bread) mixed with
⅜ cup tomato sauce (1 Vegetable)
1 corn tortilla (1 Bread)
2 cups tossed dinner salad (2 Vegetable)
2 tablespoons oil and vinegar dressing (2 Fat)

Snack

1 large orange (2 Fruit)
1 cup plain, nonfat yogurt (1 Milk)
½ cup unsweetened fruit cocktail (1 Fruit)

Week 1—Friday

Breakfast

½ cup orange juice (1 Fruit)
1½ cups cooked oatmeal or oat bran cereal without salt
   (3 Bread)
1 mashed banana (2 Fruit)
1 cup skim milk (1 Milk)

Lunch

1½ cups Long Grain and Wild Rice Chicken Salad (3
   Meat, 3 Bread, 1½ Vegetable, 1½ Fruit, 3 Fat)
   (750 mg Sodium), see p. 161, on
½ cup shredded lettuce
12 saltine crackers, unsalted tops (2 Bread)

Dinner

1 piece Vegetarian Lasagna (2 Bread, 2 Meat, 2½ Vegetable, ½ Fat) (350 mg Sodium), see p. 179
1 cup cooked green beans (2 Vegetable) with
1 teaspoon unsalted margarine (1 Fat)
1 whole wheat dinner roll (1 Bread) with
2 teaspoons unsalted margarine (2 Fat)
1 cup fresh fruit salad (2 Fruit)
½ cup skim milk (½ Milk)

Snack

1 cup raw celery sticks (1 Vegetable)
1 tablespoon cream cheese (1 Fat)

Week 1—Saturday

Breakfast

½ cup orange juice (1 Fruit)
3 slices French Toast Puff (3 Meat, ⅜ Milk, 1½ Fruit, 3
    Bread) (690 mg Sodium), see p. 154, with
2 teaspoons unsalted margarine (2 Fat) and
½ cup plain, nonfat yogurt (½ Milk) and
4 tablespoons Berry Syrup (2 Fruit) (0 mg Sodium), see
    p. 185
½ cup skim milk (½ Milk)

Lunch

½ cup Tuna Salad (2 Meat, 1 Milk) (707 mg Sodium),
    see p. 162, on
1 lettuce leaf
1 cup chopped cucumbers and tomatoes (1 Vegetable)
    mixed with
1 tablespoon oil and vinegar dressing (1 Fat)
1 large apple (3 Fruit)

Dinner

3 Stuffed Shells (1 Meat, 2 Bread, 3 Vegetable, ½ Fat)
    (150 mg Sodium), see p. 178
½ cup steamed broccoli (1 Vegetable) with
1 teaspoon unsalted margarine (1 Fat)
1 cup tossed dinner salad with cucumber and carrot
    slices (1 Vegetable)
1 tablespoon oil and vinegar dressing (1 Fat)

Snack

2 small oatmeal cookies (2 Bread)
1 cup skim milk (1 Milk)

Week 1—Sunday

Breakfast

½ grapefruit (1 Fruit)
3 Oatmeal Pancakes (3 Bread, ½ Milk) (597 mg Sodium), see p. 156
2 teaspoons unsalted margarine (2 Fat)
4 tablespoons low-calorie syrup (1 Fruit)
⅔ cup skim milk (⅔ Milk)

Lunch

1 fruit salad:
  ¾ cup fresh strawberries (1 Fruit)
  24 large green grapes (2 Fruit)
  1 sliced banana (2 Fruit)
  1 sliced small apple (1 Fruit)
¾ cup low-fat cottage cheese (3 Meat)
12 saltine crackers, unsalted tops (2 Bread)

Dinner

4 ounces Teriyaki Steak (4 Meat, ½ Vegetable, ½ Fat) (472 mg Sodium), see p. 174
1 cup steamed rice (2 Bread) with
1 teaspoon unsalted margarine (1 Fat)
2 cups stir-fry vegetables:
  ½ cup julienne zucchini (1 Vegetable)
  ½ cup julienne carrots (1 Vegetable)
  ½ cup chopped red bell pepper (1 Vegetable)
  ½ cup sliced onion (1 Vegetable)
  2 teaspoons safflower oil (2 Fat)
  ½ teaspoon ginger powder
  ½ teaspoon minced garlic

Snack

1 cup frozen yogurt (2 Milk)
1 cup unsalted pretzel sticks (2 Bread)

Week 2—Monday

Breakfast

1 cup unsweetened orange juice (2 Fruit)
2 waffles (2 Bread, 2 Fat) topped with
½ cup unsweetened applesauce (1 Fruit) and
1 teaspoon cinnamon
1 cup skim milk (1 Milk)

Lunch

3 ounces grilled tuna steak (3 Meat)
1 large baked potato (3 Bread) topped with
2 tablespoons grated cheddar cheese (½ Meat) and
2 teaspoons unsalted margarine (2 Fat)
1 cup fresh fruit salad (2 Fruit) with
¼ cup low-fat cottage cheese (1 Meat)
1 whole wheat dinner roll (1 Bread)
1 teaspoon unsalted margarine (1 Fat)

Dinner

3 ounces Grilled Sesame Chicken Breast (3 Meat, ½
    Fat, ½ Fruit) (443 mg Sodium), see p. 164
1 cup cooked corkscrew pasta (2 Bread) with
1 teaspoon unsalted margarine (1 Fat)
1 cup steamed broccoli (2 Vegetable)
1 cup marinated vegetables:
    ½ cup sliced tomato
    ½ cup sliced cucumber
    (tomato and cucumber = 1 Vegetable)
    2 tablespoons oil and vinegar dressing (2 Fat)
½ cantaloupe (2 Fruit)
1 cup skim milk (1 Milk)

Week 2—Tuesday

Breakfast

½ cup unsweetened orange juice (1 Fruit)
2 Oat Bran Muffins (1 Bread, 1 Fruit, 1 Fat) (120 mg
    Sodium), see p. 155
¼ cup scrambled egg substitute (1 Meat) cooked with
    vegetable oil cooking spray
2 teaspoons unsalted margarine (2 Fat)
1 cup skim milk (1 Milk)

Lunch

1½ cups Low-Sodium Minestrone Soup (1½ Bread, 1½
    Vegetable) (86 mg Sodium), see p. 157
1 turkey sandwich:
  2 slices whole wheat bread (2 Bread)
  4 ounces sliced turkey breast (4 Meat)
  1 teaspoon diet mayonnaise (½ Fat)
  ¼ cup alfalfa sprouts (1 Vegetable)
  1 slice tomato (½ Vegetable)
1 cup plain, nonfat yogurt (1 Milk) with
1 teaspoon sugar substitute and
1 teaspoon vanilla
¾ cup fresh strawberries (1 Fruit)
1 slice (¹⁄₂₄), angel food cake (1 Bread)

Dinner

2½ cups Low-Sodium Shrimp Creole (3 Meat, 2 Bread,
    3 Vegetable) (436 mg Sodium), see p. 171
2 3-inch slices French bread (2 Bread)
2 teaspoons unsalted margarine (2 Fat)
Lettuce wedge with
1 tablespoon French dressing (1 Fat)
1 large baked apple (3 Fruit)

Snack

3 cups air-popped popcorn (1 Bread)
1 cup apple juice (3 Fruit)

Week 2—Wednesday

Breakfast

2 English muffins (4 Bread)
2 teaspoons unsalted margarine (2 Fat)
1 fresh fruit cup:
   ½ sliced banana (1 Fruit)
   1 sliced orange (1 Fruit)
1 cup homemade cocoa:
   1 cup heated skim milk (1 Milk)
   1 tablespoon cocoa
   1 teaspoon sugar substitute

Lunch

2 tostadas:
   2 flour tortillas (2 Bread)
   ½ cup cooked, drained ground beef (2 Meat)
   2 tablespoons picante sauce
   ¼ cup grated cheddar cheese (1 Meat)
   ½ cup chopped tomato (1 Vegetable)
½ cantaloupe (2 Fruit)

Dinner

3 ounces Veal Scaloppine (3 Meat, 1½ Vegetable, 1 Fat,
   1 Bread) (252 mg Sodium), see p. 168
1 cup cooked egg noodles (2 Bread)
½ cup steamed green beans (1 Vegetable)
1 cup romaine lettuce with
1 tablespoon oil and vinegar dressing (1 Fat)
1 3-inch slice Italian Bread (1 Bread)
1 teaspoon unsalted margarine (1 Fat)
½ cup unsweetened, canned pears (1 Fruit)

Snack

1 small apple (1 Fruit)

Week 2—Thursday

Breakfast

2 Bran Muffins (2 Bread, 1 Fruit, 2 Fat) (400 mg Sodium), see p. 155
2 teaspoons unsalted margarine (2 Fat)
¼ cup scrambled egg substitute (1 Meat) cooked with vegetable oil cooking spray
½ fresh grapefruit (1 Fruit)

Lunch

2 cups cooked spaghetti (4 Bread)
1 cup Low-Sodium Italian Tomato Sauce (3 Vegetable) (40 mg Sodium), see p. 185
2 3-inch slices Italian bread (2 Bread)
2 teaspoons unsalted margarine (2 Fat)
1 small fresh peach (1 Fruit)

Dinner

1 serving Low-Sodium Beef Broccoli Stir-Fry (4 Meat, 2 Vegetable, ½ Fat) (544 mg Sodium), see p. 172
¾ cup cooked rice (1½ Bread)
1 oriental salad:
  1 cup mixed greens
  ½ cup unsweetened mandarin oranges (1 Fruit)
  1 tablespoon slivered almonds (1 Fat)
  1 tablespoon oil and vinegar dressing (1 Fat)
1 cup Apple Oat Crisp (2 Fruit, 1 Bread, ½ Fat) (80 mg Sodium), see p. 180
1 cup skim milk (1 Milk)

Snack

¼ cup low-fat cottage cheese (1 Meat)
½ cup unsweetened, canned pears (1 Fruit)

Week 2—Friday

Breakfast

1 cup unsweetened grapefruit juice (2 Fruit)
1½ cups corn bran cereal (2 Bread)
½ cup fresh blueberries (1 Fruit)
1 cup skim milk (1 Milk)
1 slice whole wheat toast (1 Bread)
1 teaspoon unsalted margarine (1 Fat)

Lunch

2 servings Low-Sodium Seafood Quiche (1 Milk, 5
    Meat) (700 mg Sodium), see p. 170
½ cup steamed asparagus (1 Vegetable)
½ cup Apple Waldorf Salad (1 Fruit, 1 Fat) (76 mg So-
    dium), see p. 159
2 whole wheat dinner rolls (2 Bread)

Dinner

2 tacos:
    2 taco shells (1 Bread, 1 Fat)
    ½ cup cooked, seasoned ground chicken (2 Meat)
    ¼ cup chopped tomato (½ Vegetable)
    shredded lettuce
    picante sauce
1 cup steamed zucchini (2 Vegetable)
1 cup sugar-free vanilla pudding (1 Milk) with
1 sliced banana (2 Fruit) and
8 vanilla wafers (2 Bread)

Snack

1 chicken sandwich:
    2 slices rye bread (2 Bread)
    ¼ cup cooked, diced chicken (1 meat)
    1 small chopped apple (1 Fruit)
    3 teaspoons diet mayonnaise (1 Fat)
½ cup unsweetened orange juice (1 Fruit)

Week 2—Saturday

Breakfast

1 cup unsweetened orange juice (2 Fruit)
2 large shredded wheat biscuits (2 Bread)
1 slice whole wheat toast (1 Bread)
1 teaspoon unsalted margarine (1 Fat)
1 cup skim milk (1 Milk)

Lunch

1½ servings Ricotta-Parmesan Torte (1½ Fat, 1 Vegetable, 2 Bread, 1½ Meat) (547 mg Sodium), see p. 175
2 4-inch breadsticks (1 Bread)
1 cup steamed, mixed vegetables (2 Vegetable)
1 teaspoon unsalted margarine (1 Fat)
½ cup Turkey-Fruit Salad (1 Meat, 1 Fruit, ½ Vegetable) (75 mg Sodium), see p. 163
12 large green grapes (1 Fruit)

Dinner

3 ounces Low-Sodium Southern Fried Chicken (3 Meat, ½ Bread, ½ Fat) (195 mg Sodium), see p. 165
1½ cups mashed potatoes (3 Bread)
½ cup steamed French-cut green beans (1 Vegetable)
1 cup fresh pineapple (2 Fruit)
2 teaspoons unsalted margarine (2 Fat)

Snack

1 cup skim milk (1 Milk)
8 vanilla wafers (2 Bread)
1 small fresh peach (1 Fruit)

Week 2—Sunday

Breakfast

1 cup unsweetened grapefruit juice (2 Fruit)
1 English muffin (2 Bread) topped with
1 small sliced apple (1 Fruit) and
2 tablespoons grated cheddar cheese (½ Meat)
1½ cups bran flakes (2 Bread)
1 cup skim milk (1 Milk)

Lunch

1 chicken salad sandwich:
   2 slices whole wheat bread (2 Bread)
   ½ cup cooked, chopped chicken (2 Meat)
   2 tablespoons diet mayonnaise (2 Fat)
   ¼ cup chopped celery (½ Vegetable)
6 raw carrot sticks (1 Vegetable)
1 small fresh pear (1 Fruit)

Dinner

4 ounces Shishkabob (4 Meat, 3 Vegetable) (392 mg
    Sodium), see p. 173
1 medium baked potato (2 Bread) with
1 tablespoon sour cream (1 Fat) and
2 teaspoons unsalted margarine and
1 teaspoon chives
½ cup steamed broccoli (1 Vegetable)
¼ honeydew melon (2 Fruit)

Snack

1 cup plain, nonfat yogurt (1 Milk)
½ cup frozen or fresh unsweetened raspberries (1
    Fruit)

Recipes: The Antihypertensive Meal Plan

Breakfasts

Bran Muffins

Yields: 14 muffins
1 serving (1 muffin):

Calories	*= 127*	*Exchanges = 1 Bread +*	
Cholesterol	*= 18 mg*	*½ Fruit +*	
Fat	*= 5 gm*	*1 Fat*	
Sodium	*= 200 mg*		

¾ cup all-purpose flour
½ cup whole wheat flour
1 tablespoon baking powder
½ teaspoon "lite" salt
¼ cup sugar
2½ cups bran flakes cereal
1¼ cups skim milk
1 egg
¼ cup safflower oil

Preheat oven to 400° F. Stir together flour, baking powder, salt, and sugar. Set aside. Measure bran flakes and milk into large mixing bowl. Let stand 1 to 2 minutes while cereal softens. Add egg and oil. Beat well. Add flour mixture. Stir only until combined. Spoon batter evenly into 14 greased muffin tins. Bake for 18 to 20 minutes or until done.

French Toast Puff

Yields: 4 servings
1 serving (1 slice):

Calories	*= 215*	*Exchanges =*	*1 Meat +*
Cholesterol	*= 2 mg*		*1 Bread +*
Fat	*= 8 gm*		*½ Fruit +*
Sodium	*= 230 mg*		*⅛ Milk*

1 cup egg substitute
½ cup evaporated skimmed milk
1 tablespoon honey
½ teaspoon ground cinnamon
¼ teaspoon ground mace
4 1-ounce slices cinnamon-raisin bread, cut diagonally in half
   nonstick vegetable cooking spray

Preheat oven to 350 °F. Spray a 9-inch pie plate with cooking spray. In medium bowl, whisk together all ingredients except bread. Place bread in prepared plate; pour milk mixture over bread. Cover with plastic wrap and refrigerate at least 1 hour or overnight. Bake 25 to 30 minutes, until puffy and golden brown. Serve at once.

Optional:
Sprinkle with confectioner's sugar or Berry Syrup, see p. 185

Oat Bran Muffins

Yields: 24 1-inch muffins
1 serving (1 muffin):

Calories	*= 66*	*Exchanges = ½ Bread +*
Cholesterol	*= 0 mg*	*½ Fruit +*
Fat	*= 1 gm*	*½ Fat*
Sodium	*= 60 mg*	

1¼ cups oat bran cereal
  1 cup whole wheat flour
  ⅓ cup raisins
  1 tablespoon baking powder
  ½ cup skim milk
  ½ cup unsweetened orange juice
  ¼ cup honey
  2 tablespoons safflower oil
  3 egg whites

Preheat oven to 425° F. Mix together dry ingredients. Add skim milk, orange juice, honey, oil, and egg whites. Mix. Divide mixture into mini-muffin tins. Bake for 15 minutes or until lightly browned.

Oatmeal Pancakes

Yields: 12 5-inch diameter pancakes
1 serving (1 pancake):

Calories	= 98	Exchanges = 1 Bread +
Cholesterol	= 1 mg	⅙ Milk
Fat	= 1 gm	
Sodium	= 199 mg	

1½ cups uncooked oatmeal
 2 cups buttermilk
 2 egg whites
 1 cup whole wheat flour
 2 teaspoons baking soda
 1 mashed banana

Combine oatmeal, buttermilk, and egg whites and let stand for at least ½ hour or refrigerate up to 24 hours. Add remaining ingredients and stir the batter just until the dry ingredients are moistened. Cook on each side on a hot, lightly oiled griddle.

Soups

Gazpacho

Yields: 6 servings
1 serving (¾ cup):
Calories   = 60
Cholesterol = 0 mg
Fat   = 3 gm
Sodium   = 24 mg

Exchanges = 1½ Vegetable +
½ Fat

4 cups low-sodium tomato juice
½ cup unpeeled chopped cucumber
¼ cup chopped green pepper
¼ cup finely chopped onion
1 tablespoon olive oil
2 tablespoons wine vinegar
½ teaspoon pepper
1 teaspoon dried oregano
2 teaspoons chopped fresh basil
1 minced garlic clove

Combine all ingredients. Cover and chill overnight.

Minestrone Soup

Yields: 8 servings
1 serving (1 cup):
Calories   = 100
Cholesterol = 0 mg
Fat   = 1 gm
Sodium   = 170 mg

Exchanges = 1 Bread +
1 Vegetable

         1 diced onion
      1½ cups chopped celery
       ¼ cup homemade vegetable stock or low-sodium
           broth
*14½- or 16-ounce can tomatoes with juice
         3 cups homemade vegetable stock or low-sodium
           broth
         3 cups water
       ¼ cup chopped parsley
           dash of pepper
         2 bay leaves
         1 teaspoon oregano
         2 teaspoons basil
       ½ teaspoon rosemary
         1 minced garlic clove
       ½ cup chopped carrot
       ½ cup diced zucchini
       ½ cup diced potato
       ¼ cup chopped green pepper
       ¼ cup fresh frozen corn
         1 cup sliced fresh mushrooms
       ½ cup uncooked spaghetti
         1 cup canned and rinsed garbanzo beans
       ½ cup cooked barley

Sauté onion and celery in vegetable stock until soft. Add
the tomatoes, vegetable stock, water, parsley, seasonings, and vegetables. Simmer soup for 30 minutes. Add
spaghetti, garbanzo beans, and cooked barley. Continue
cooking over medium heat for 10 minutes.

*Lower-Sodium Variation:
  Substitute low-sodium canned tomatoes.
  1 serving: Sodium =57 mg

Salads

Apple Waldorf Salad

Yields: 4 servings
1 serving (½ cup):

Calories	*= 90*
Cholesterol	*= 0 mg*
Fat	*= 4 gm*
Sodium	*= 76 mg*

Exchanges = 1 Fruit +
1 Fat

  1 chopped Granny Smith apple
  1 chopped red delicious apple
  1 tablespoon fresh lemon juice
  ½ cup chopped celery
  1 tablespoon coarsely chopped pecan halves
  ¼ cup plain, nonfat yogurt
     dash ground cinnamon
     dash ground nutmeg
  2 tablespoons diet mayonnaise

Sprinkle apples with lemon juice. Add all other ingredients and combine gently. Serve on purple cabbage leaf or lettuce leaf.

Cold Pasta Salad

Yields: 4 servings
1 serving (1 cup):

Calories	*= 240*	*Exchanges = 1½ Bread +*
Cholesterol	*= 14 mg*	*½ Meat +*
Fat	*= 7 gm*	*2 Vegetable +*
Sodium	*= 412 mg*	*½ Fat*

        6 ounces (3 cups) cooked pasta
    *½ cup feta cheese
    *⅓ cup low-calorie Italian dressing
      ¼ cup chopped green onion
        2 tablespoons sliced, pitted black olives
6 to 8 cherry tomatoes, cut in half
        6 cups fresh spinach, washed and stems cut

Combine all ingredients except spinach. Arrange spinach on serving platter and arrange pasta salad on top.

Lower-Sodium Variation:
  Substitute part-skim mozzarella cheese and vinegar and oil dressing.
  1 serving:
  Calories   = 265
  Cholesterol = 8 mg
  Fat   = 10 gm
  Sodium   = 163 mg

Long Grain and Wild Rice Chicken Salad

Yields: 10 servings
1 serving (½ cup):
Calories = 260
Cholesterol = 30 mg
Fat = 11 gm
Sodium = 250 mg

Exchanges = 1 *Meat* +
1 *Bread* +
1 *Fat* +
½ *Vegetable* +
½ *Fruit*

¾ cup uncooked long grain brown rice
¼ cup uncooked wild rice
2½ cups water
½ cup diet mayonnaise
½ cup skim milk
½ cup lemon juice
1 small (¼ cup) grated onion
1 teaspoon chopped chives
12 ounces cooked chicken, cubed
1 can (8 ounces) drained and chopped water chestnuts
½ teaspoon curry powder
½ teaspoon pepper
½ pound seedless green grapes, cut in half
½ cup chopped nuts (optional)

Combine rice and water in saucepan and heat to boiling.
Lower heat and cover. Simmer 1 hour or until tender.
Combine mayonnaise, milk, lemon juice, onion, and chives
in large bowl, blending well. Stir in chicken, water chestnuts, curry powder, and pepper, mixing well. Stir in
cooked rice. Refrigerate two hours or until chilled. At
serving time, fold in halved grapes. Spoon salad on serving
platter, lined with lettuce. Top with chopped nuts, if
desired.

Tuna Salad

Yields: 2 servings
1 serving (½ cup):
Calories   = 190   *Exchanges = 2 Meat +*
Cholesterol = 65 mg   *1 Milk*
Fat   = 2 gm
Sodium   = 707 mg

6½-ounce can (1 cup) water-packed, low-sodium tuna,
  drained
4 teaspoons diet Miracle Whip
4 tablespoons plain, low-fat yogurt
2 cooked, chopped egg whites
*½ chopped dill pickle
  onion powder, to taste
  pepper, to taste
1 to 2 tablespoons chopped apple (optional)

Combine all ingredients and mix well.

Lower-Sodium Variation:
 Omit dill pickle.
 1 serving: Sodium = 225 mg

Turkey-Fruit Salad

Yields: 4 servings
1 serving (1 cup):

Calories	*= 185*
Cholesterol	*= 30 mg*
Fat	*= 4 gm*
Sodium	*= 150 mg*

Exchanges = ½ Meat +
2 Fruit +
1 Vegetable

⅓ cup plain, low-fat yogurt
 1 tablespoon diet mayonnaise
 1 tablespoon honey
½ teaspoon finely shredded orange peel
⅛ teaspoon salt
 1 cup cooked, cubed turkey
 1 cup halved fresh strawberries
 1 small banana, cut in ½-inch slices
½ cup sliced celery
 2 medium peeled and sliced oranges
    lettuce leaves

Blend first five ingredients together and set aside. Combine remaining ingredients in a separate bowl. Fold the first mixture into the salad ingredients. Chill.

Main Courses

Grilled Sesame Chicken Breasts

Yields: 4 servings
1 serving (4 ounces):

Calories	*= 265*	*Exchanges = 3½ Meat +*
Cholesterol	*= 73 mg*	*½ Fruit +*
Fat	*= 11 gm*	*1 Fat +*
Sodium	*= 590 mg*	*½ Bread*

½ cup unsweetened white grape juice
¼ cup low-sodium "lite" soy sauce
¼ cup dry white wine
1 tablespoon sesame seeds
2 tablespoons safflower oil
¼ teaspoon garlic powder
¼ teaspoon ground ginger
1 teaspoon liquid smoke flavoring
16 ounces skinless, boneless chicken breasts

Combine all ingredients except chicken in a shallow dish; mix well. Add chicken, turning to coat; cover and marinate in refrigerator at least 4 hours. Remove chicken from marinade, reserving marinade. Grill 4 to 5 inches from medium-hot flame or coals for 15 minutes, turning and basting frequently with marinade.

Southern Fried Chicken

Yields: 6 servings
1 serving (⅙ recipe):

Calories	*= 262*	*Exchanges =*	*4 Meat +*
Cholesterol	*= 101 mg*		*½ Bread +*
Fat	*= 11 gm*		*½ Fat*
Sodium	*= 260 mg*		

24 ounces skinless, boneless chicken
 1 tablespoon safflower oil
⅓ cup white flour
*1 teaspoon "lite" salt
½ teaspoon paprika
¼ teaspoon poultry seasoning
¼ teaspoon garlic powder
⅛ teaspoon pepper
½ cup water

Select a large nonstick skillet with a closely fitting lid. Remove all skin and visible fat from chicken. Combine flour and spices in plastic bag or bowl. Shake or roll chicken, one or two pieces at a time in seasoned flour. Set aside on waxed paper. Coat all chicken with flour before heating oil. Heat 1 tablespoon oil in the skillet, then add chicken. Brown over medium heat, about 10 to 12 minutes per side, until golden brown on all sides. Add ½ cup water to chicken. Cover tightly, cook over low heat for 30 minutes. Remove cover, turn up heat, and cook off any remaining liquid. Continue frying chicken until reddish-brown, 1 to 2 minutes.

Lower-Sodium Variation:
 Omit "lite" salt.
 1 serving: Sodium = 98 mg

Spanish Chicken and Rice

Yields: 2 servings
1 serving (1 cup):

Calories	*= 421*	*Exchanges = 3½ Meat +*
Cholesterol	*= 75 mg*	*2 Bread +*
Fat	*= 12 gm*	*2 Vegetable +*
Sodium	*= 375 mg*	*1 Fat*

  2 teaspoons olive oil
  ½ cup diced onion
  ½ cup chopped green pepper
  2 minced garlic cloves
  ½ cup canned low-sodium tomato sauce
  ⅓ cup water
  ½ cup low-sodium chicken broth
  ¼ teaspoon ground cumin
     dash pepper
  6 ounces cooked skinless, boneless chicken
  1 cup cooked long grain rice
  2 ounces cooked pinto beans
  1 tablespoon chopped fresh parsley

In a 10-inch skillet, heat oil; then add onion, green pepper,
and garlic. Sauté over low heat until tender, about 5
minutes. Add tomato sauce, water, broth, and seasonings
and bring to a boil. Reduce heat and let simmer 5 minutes;
stir in remaining ingredients and cook until thoroughly
heated.

Peppered Veal

Yields: 6 servings
1 serving (2½ ounces):

Calories   = 225
Cholesterol = 58 mg   *Exchanges* = 2½ *Meat* +
Fat   = 12 gm   1 *Vegetable* +
Sodium   = 208 mg   ½ *Bread* +
                                         ½ *Fat*

  1 pound veal cutlets
  ¼ teaspoon freshly ground pepper
  1 crushed garlic clove
  2 teaspoons olive oil
  1 medium onion, cut into strips
  2 green peppers, seeded and cut into strips
  ½ cup dry white wine
  ½ cup water
*1 teaspoon beef-flavored bouillon granules
  ½ teaspoon dried whole basil
  ¼ teaspoon dried whole oregano
1½ teaspoons cornstarch
  2 tablespoons water
12 cherry tomatoes, cut in half

Trim excess fat from veal cutlets; cut into 1-inch strips. Sprinkle with pepper. Sauté garlic in olive oil in a large skillet over medium-high heat until tender. Add cutlets and cook until browned. Stir in next 7 ingredients and bring to a boil. Cover; reduce heat and simmer 5 minutes or until vegetables are crisp-tender. Combine cornstarch and water, stirring until blended; stir into veal mixture. Bring to a boil and cook 1 minute or until slightly thickened. Stir in tomatoes. Serve over corkscrew pasta, rice, or noodles.

Lower-Sodium Variation:
  Substitute low-sodium bouillon granules
  1 serving: Sodium = 50 mg

Veal Scaloppine

Yields: 4 servings
1 serving (3 ounces):

Calories	*= 290*	*Exchanges = 3 Meat +*
Cholesterol	*= 65 mg*	*1½ Vegetable +*
Fat	*= 15 gm*	*1 Fat +*
Sodium	*= 252 mg*	*1 Bread*

    8 ounces (2 cups) sliced fresh mushrooms
  ⅛ teaspoon pepper
  ½ cup dry white wine
  12 ounces (4 3-ounce pieces) veal scaloppine
    2 tablespoons flour
    1 tablespoon olive oil
  ¾ cup minced onion
    1 cup chicken broth

Place mushrooms, pepper and wine in a small saucepan.
Simmer uncovered for about 10 minutes until mushrooms
are tender. Pound the veal with flat side of meat mallet or
with a rolling pin to half the original thickness. Sprinkle
with "lite" salt, if desired, then dredge with flour. Heat
olive oil in a large nonstick skillet over high heat. Add
onion and shake pan to distribute onion evenly. Arrange
breaded cutlets on bed of onion in skillet and cook for 1 or
2 minutes over high heat until meat begins to brown. Turn
and cook for 1 or 2 minutes to brown other side. Reduce
heat to low, add broth, and simmer for 2 minutes. Turn
veal and add the mushroom mixture. Increase the heat and
cook for 3 to 5 minutes until fluid is reduced and sauce is
slightly thickened.

Variation:
Turkey Scaloppine: Substitute turkey cutlets (sliced raw
breast meat) for veal.

Herbed Garlic Fish Fillets
(microwave recipe)

Yields: 4 servings
1 serving (3 ounces):
Calories   = 146   *Exchanges = 3 Meat*
Cholesterol = 47 mg
Fat   = 6 gm
Sodium   = 202 mg

  1 tablespoon water
  1 teaspoon grated orange peel
 ½ teaspoon crushed dried rosemary leaves
 ¼ teaspoon crushed dried thyme leaves
  1 minced garlic clove
 ¼ cup chopped fresh parsley
 12 ounces fish fillets, about ½ inch thick, cut into 4
     serving-size pieces

In a small ceramic bowl, combine water, orange peel, rosemary, thyme, and garlic. Cover with plastic wrap. Microwave at HIGH for 1 minute. Stir in parsley. Arrange fillets in a 9-inch square baking dish with thickest portions toward outside of dish. Top with parsley mixture. Cover with wax paper. Microwave at HIGH for 5 to 7 minutes, or until fish flakes easily with fork, rotating dish once. Let stand, covered, for 3 minutes.

Seafood Quiche

Yields: 8 servings
1 serving (⅛ of quiche):

Calories	= 185	*Exchanges* = ½ Milk +
Cholesterol	= 70 mg	2½ Meat
Fat	= 7 gm	
Sodium	= 475 mg	

   2 eggs or equivalent egg substitute
   4 egg whites, beaten well
   6 ounces precooked shrimp
 *6 ounces crab meat
   2 chopped green onions
10 to 12 (about 4 ounces) thinly sliced medium mushrooms
 1¼ cup evaporated skimmed milk
   2 cups grated part-skim mozzarella cheese
    nonstick vegetable cooking spray

Preheat oven to 350° F. Mix all ingredients and pour into a 9-inch pan sprayed with nonstick vegetable cooking spray. Bake for 30 to 40 minutes until firm and lightly browned.

Lower-Sodium Variation:
Omit crab and add 6 ounces more shrimp.
1 serving:

Calories	= 169
Cholesterol	= 77 mg
Fat	= 5 gm
Sodium	= 350 mg

Shrimp Creole

Yields: 6 servings
1 serving (1¾ cup):

Calories = 282	*Exchanges* = 2 Meat +
Cholesterol = 106 mg	*1½ Bread* +
Fat = 3 gm	*2 Vegetable*
Sodium = 450 mg	

  2 tablespoons diet margarine
  ½ cup diced onion
  ½ cup diced celery
  ½ cup diced green pepper
  1 minced garlic clove
  2 8-ounce cans low-sodium tomato sauce
  ⅛ teaspoon pepper
  ¼ teaspoon chili powder
*¾ teaspoon "lite" salt
  1 pound cooked shrimp, cut in pieces
  4 cups cooked rice

Melt margarine in skillet. Sauté vegetables and garlic in melted margarine. Blend together tomato sauce, pepper, chili powder and "lite" salt. Add tomato mixture to vegetables and simmer for 15 minutes. Add cooked shrimp and heat thoroughly. Serve over cooked rice.

Lower-Sodium Variation:
  Omit "lite" salt.
  1 serving: Sodium = 291 mg

Beef Broccoli Stir-Fry

Yields: 4 servings
1 serving (¼ recipe):
Calories   = 349   *Exchanges = 4 Meat +*
Cholesterol = 76 mg   *2 Vegetable +*
Fat   = 13 gm   *½ Fat*
Sodium   = 736 mg

1 pound lean flank steak or top round, trimmed of fat
1 large bunch (approximately 2 pounds) fresh broccoli
2 teaspoons safflower oil
2 minced garlic cloves
2 tablespoons water

Marinade
   2 teaspoons sake (rice wine) or cooking sherry
 ½ teaspoon baking soda
   2 tablespoons low-sodium "lite" soy sauce
1½ teaspoons cornstarch
   2 teaspoons safflower oil
 ½ teaspoon sugar
 ½ teaspoon ground ginger

Sauce
   2 teaspoons cornstarch
*1 cup beef broth
   1 teaspoon low-sodium "lite" soy sauce·
 ¼ to ½ teaspoon pepper

Trim beef of all fat, then slice across the grain into ⅛-inch
strips. Combine marinade ingredients in medium bowl.
Add beef strips and mix well. Let stand 20 to 30 minutes
to tenderize. Trim tough stems and leaves from broccoli.
Break tops into bite-sized florets and cut stems into
½-inch slices. Combine sauce ingredients in small bowl

and set aside. Heat a large nonstick skillet or wok until very hot. Add beef strips with marinade. Stir-fry over highest possible heat until lightly browned. Remove beef from skillet and set aside. Heat the 2 teaspoons safflower oil in the same skillet. Add minced garlic and prepare broccoli. Stir-fry over high heat for 3 to 5 minutes until broccoli is crisp-tender. Add water, cover tightly, and steam over medium heat for 3 minutes. Remove lid. Add sauce ingredients. Stir until sauce bubbles. Add beef, heat through, and serve immediately.

Lower-Sodium Variation:
Substitute low-sodium beef broth.
1 serving: Sodium = 544 mg

Shishkabob

4 servings
Per serving (3 ounces meat):

Calories	= 257	Exchanges = 3 Meat +
Cholesterol	= 60 mg	2 Vegetable
Fat	= 9 gm	
Sodium	= 295 mg	

1 pound lean meat (flank), cut in chunks and trimmed of fat
½ cup commercial oil-free Italian salad dressing
½ cup red wine
8 cherry tomatoes
½ medium onion, cut in 8 chunks
½ green pepper, cut in 8 chunks
1 zucchini, cut in 8 chunks
4 skewers

Marinate meat overnight in salad dressing and wine, turning once. On each skewer, alternate ¼ of the meat chunks, 2 cherry tomatoes, 2 chunks of onion, 2 chunks of green pepper, and 2 chunks of zucchini. On a charcoal grill or in an oven broiler, cook shishkabobs 10 to 15 minutes each side, turning as needed to cook evenly throughout.

Teriyaki Steak

Yields: 6 servings
1 serving (4 ounces):

Calories	*= 280*	*Exchanges = 4 Meat +*
Cholesterol	*= 76 mg*	*½ Fat +*
Fat	*= 10 gm*	*½ Vegetable*
Sodium	*= 472 mg*	

1½ pounds lean flank steak, trimmed of fat
 1 tablespoon olive oil
 ¼ cup low-sodium "lite" soy sauce
 ¼ cup pineapple juice
 2 tablespoons vinegar
1½ teaspoons ground ginger
 2 tablespoons finely chopped green onion
 1 minced garlic clove
 1 tablespoon cooking sherry

Trim excess fat from steak. Score steak with ⅛-inch deep diagonal cuts on both sides. Combine remaining ingredients in large, shallow dish; add steak, turning to coat well with marinade. Cover and marinate in refrigerator 4 hours or overnight, turning occasionally. Remove steak from marinade. Broil steak 4 to 5 inches from heat, 5 to 7 minutes on each side or until desired degree of doneness. Transfer steak to a cutting board; cut in thin slices across grain.

Note: May also be cooked over hot coals.

Ricotta-Parmesan Torte

Yields: 8 servings
1 serving (1 piece):

Calories	*= 250*	*Exchanges =*	*1 Fat +*
Cholesterol	*= 144 mg*		*½ Vegetable +*
Fat	*= 12 gm*		*1½ Bread +*
Sodium	*= 365 mg*		*1 Meat*

Dough
¾ cup all-purpose white flour
3 tablespoons warm water
1 tablespoon plus 1 teaspoon safflower oil
⅛ teaspoon salt

Filling
1 tablespoon plus 1 teaspoon margarine
1 cup minced scallions (green onion)
1 cup grated zucchini
½ cup grated carrots
2 minced garlic cloves
2 cups cooked long-grain rice
1 cup part-skim ricotta cheese
4 eggs (or 8 egg whites)
3 tablespoons grated part-skim Parmesan cheese, divided
⅛ teaspoon salt
⅛ teaspoon freshly ground pepper

To Prepare Dough:
In a small mixing bowl, combine flour, water, oil, and salt. Using your hands, knead dough into a smooth ball (dough should hold together but not be sticky; if necessary, add up to 1 more tablespoon warm water to adjust consistency). Wrap dough in plastic wrap and set aside while preparing filling (plastic wrap will prevent dough from cracking).

To Prepare Filling:
In a 10-inch nonstick skillet, heat margarine until bubbly and hot. Add vegetables and garlic and sauté over medium-low heat, stirring occasionally until vegetables are soft, about 3 minutes. Set aside and let cool. In large mixing bowl, combine rice, ricotta cheese, 3 eggs, 2 tablespoons Parmesan cheese, salt and pepper; beat until smooth. Add cooled vegetables and stir to combine.

To Prepare Torte:
Preheat oven to 350° F. Between 2 sheets of wax paper roll dough, forming a rectangle about ⅛ inch thick. Remove paper and lift dough into a 10 x 6 x 2-inch baking dish so that edges of dough extend slightly over sides of dish. Spoon cheese mixture over dough and bring up sides of dough over edges of filling, leaving center uncovered. In small bowl, beat remaining egg with remaining tablespoon Parmesan cheese. Pour over entire surface of torte. Bake until brown, about 1 hour. Remove from oven and let stand until set, about 15 minutes. Serve warm or at room temperature.

Spicy Bean Enchiladas

Yields: 8 servings
1 serving (1 enchilada):

Calories	*= 200*	*Exchanges = 1 Meat +*	
Cholesterol	*= 3 mg*	*2 Bread +*	
Fat	*= 2 gm*	*½ Vegetable*	
Sodium	*= 553 mg*		

 ¾ pound dried pinto beans
 8 cups water
 2 minced garlic cloves
 1 bay leaf
*¾ teaspoon salt
 1 recipe Spicy Tomato Sauce, see p. 187
 ½ teaspoon chili powder

¼ teaspoon pepper
8 6-inch corn tortillas
  nonstick vegetable cooking spray
1 cup (4 ounces) shredded low-fat cheddar cheese
½ cup plain, low-fat yogurt
2 tablespoons chopped green onion
  shredded lettuce (optional)

Sort and wash beans. Cover with water 2 inches above top of beans and let stand 8 hours; drain. Preheat oven to 350° F. Combine beans, 8 cups water, garlic, bay leaf, and salt in Dutch oven; bring to a boil. Cover, reduce heat to medium, and cook 1½ hours or until tender. Drain and discard bay leaf. Mash beans; add ½ cup Spicy Tomato Sauce, chili powder, and pepper, stirring well. Spread ½ cup bean mixture over each tortilla. Roll up; place seam-side down in a 13 x 9 x 2-inch baking dish coated with cooking spray. Spoon remaining Spicy Tomato Sauce over tortillas; cover and bake for 20 minutes. Top with cheese and bake uncovered an additional 5 minutes or until cheese melts. Serve with a spoonful of yogurt for each serving and sprinkle with green onions. Garnish with lettuce, if desired.

Note: If corn tortillas crack or are hard to roll up, soften by steaming. To steam, place 2 or 3 tortillas at a time in a strainer, and place over boiling water. Cover and steam 2 to 3 minutes or until softened and pliable.

*Lower-Sodium Variation:
 Omit salt.
 1 serving: Sodium = 354 mg

Stuffed Shells

Yields: 7 servings
1 serving (3 shells):

Calories	*= 320*	*Exchanges = 2 Bread +*
Cholesterol	*= 55 mg*	*3 Vegetable +*
Fat	*= 9 gm*	*1 Meat +*
Sodium	*= 150 mg*	*½ Fat*

¾ of a 12-ounce package large shells, cooked according to
   package directions (21 shells)
1 box (10 ounces) frozen chopped spinach
1 tablespoon chopped onion
2 teaspoons diet margarine
2 beaten egg whites
⅔ cup part-skim ricotta cheese
½ cup grated Parmesan cheese
½ teaspoon ground nutmeg
1 recipe Original Tomato Sauce, see p. 186

Preheat oven to 350° F. Defrost and squeeze excess
water from spinach. In skillet, cook onion in margarine
until tender. Add spinach; heat through. Combine eggs,
ricotta cheese, Parmesan cheese, nutmeg, and spinach
mixture. Pour half the sauce in a baking dish. Stuff shells
with filling. Arrange in dish and top with remaining sauce.
Bake for 30 minutes.

Vegetarian Lasagna

Yields: 8 servings
1 serving (1 piece):
Calories = 350
Cholesterol = 50 mg
Fat = 11 gm
Sodium = 350 mg

Exchanges = 2 Bread +
2 Meat +
2½ Vegetable +
½ Fat

 1 large chopped onion
 2 minced garlic cloves
 ¼ pound sliced, fresh mushrooms
 4 medium diced eggplant (or zucchini)
 1 8-ounce package lasagna noodles, cooked according to
   package directions
 1 recipe Original Tomato Sauce, see p. 186
 2 cups low-fat cottage cheese
 8 ounces grated part-skim mozzarella cheese
 ½ cup grated Parmesan cheese
 1 tablespoon safflower oil

Preheat oven to 350° F. Sauté onion and garlic in oil in
nonstick skillet until soft. Add mushrooms and eggplant (or
zucchini). Cook lasagna noodles. Mix vegetable mixture
with sautéd tomato sauce. Mix 5½ ounces mozzarella
cheese with Parmesan cheese, reserving 1½ ounces. To
prepare lasagna, layer ½ noodles on bottom of 13 x 9-inch
casserole dish; then ½ vegetable mixture; then cheese,
repeat. Sprinkle the reserved 1½ ounces of cheeses
mixture over top; then sprinkle with Parmesan cheese to
complete. Bake for 45 minutes.

Side Dishes

Apple Oat Crisp

Yields: 4 servings
1 serving (1 cup):
Calories   = 165   *Exchanges = 1 Bread +*
Cholesterol = 0 mg   *2 Fruit +*
Fat   = 3 gm   *½ Fat*
Sodium   = 80 mg

Fruit
   3 small cored and sliced apples
   ½ cup unsweetened applesauce
1½ teaspoons lemon juice
   ½ teaspoon grated lemon rind
   1 teaspoon sugar
   ¼ teaspoon ground cinnamon

Topping
   1 ounce quick-cooking oats
   2 tablespoons whole wheat flour
   2 tablespoons firmly packed brown sugar
   ¼ teaspoon ground cinnamon
   1 tablespoon plus 1 teaspoon diet margarine

Preheat oven to 350° F. In medium non-aluminum bowl, combine all fruit ingredients. Pour into an 8-inch baking dish. Prepare topping in a small bowl by combining oats, flour, brown sugar, and cinnamon. Cut margarine into topping mixture with a pastry blender until crumbly. Sprinkle topping evenly over apple mixture. Bake for 35 to 40 minutes until apples are tender and topping is browned. Serve hot.

Optional:
Top each with ½ cup ice milk.
1 serving with ½ cup ice milk:

Calories	= 260	Exchanges =	1 Milk +
Cholesterol	= 13 mg		1 Bread +
Fat	= 6 gm		2 Fruit +
Sodium	= 145 mg		½ Fat

Fruit Smoothy

Yields: 4 servings
1 serving (1 cup):

Calories	*= 100*	*Exchanges = *	*1½ Milk*
Cholesterol	*= 4 mg*		
Fat	*= 0 gm*		
Sodium	*= 85 mg*		

1 8-ounce can "lite" fruit cocktail, chilled
1 cup skim milk
¼ cup nonfat dry powdered milk
¼ cup plain, low-fat yogurt
½ teaspoon vanilla
½ cup ice cubes (3 to 4 large ice cubes)
    few dashes ground cinnamon
1 package sugar substitute (optional)

In a blender container, combine undrained fruit cocktail and remaining ingredients except the ice cubes and the cinnamon. Cover and blend until combined. Add ice cubes; cover and blend until smooth. Sprinkle with cinnamon. Serve immediately.

Italian Rice and Peas

Yields: 8 servings
1 serving (½ cup):

Calories	*= 134*	*Exchanges = 1½ Bread +*
Cholesterol	*= 3 mg*	*½ Fat*
Fat	*= 2 gm*	
Sodium	*= 206 mg*	

  1 tablespoon diet margarine
  1 small chopped onion
  1 10-ounce package frozen peas
  2 cups water
  1 cup uncooked rice
*1 teaspoon instant chicken bouillon granules
 ¼ cup grated Parmesan cheese

In a 2-quart saucepan, heat margarine, stir in onion, and cook until tender. Stir in remaining ingredients except cheese. Heat to boiling, stirring once or twice. Cover, reduce heat, and simmer 14 minutes. (Do NOT lift cover or stir). Remove from heat. Fluff rice lightly with fork; cover and let steam 5 to 10 minutes. Stir in cheese lightly with fork.

*Lower-Sodium Variation:
  Substitute low-sodium bouillon cube.
  1 serving: Sodium = 87 mg

Oven French Fries

Yields: 6 servings
1 serving (½ cup):
Calories   = 100   *Exchanges = 2 Bread*
Cholesterol = 0 mg
Fat   = 0 gm
Sodium   = 5 mg

3 to 4 (about 1 pound) thinly sliced medium baking pota-
        toes
        nonstick vegetable cooking spray
  ¼ cup minced chives
  3 tablespoons minced fresh parsley
  ½ teaspoon pepper
  ½ teaspoon paprika
  1 teaspoon minced rosemary

Preheat oven to 350° F. Layer ⅓ of potatoes in an 8-inch
square baking pan, coated with cooking spray. Sprinkle
with ⅓ of chives, parsley, pepper, paprika, and rosemary.
Repeat layers until all ingredients are used. Cover with
foil. Bake for 45 minutes or until done.

Pita Crackers

Yields: 32 crackers
1 serving (1 cracker):
Calories   = 10   *Exchanges = ⅛ Bread*
Cholesterol = 0 mg
Fat   = 0 gm
Sodium   = 23 mg

whole wheat pita pockets
nonstick vegetable cooking spray

Preheat oven to 300° F. Spray baking sheet with nonstick cooking spray. Cut 4 1-ounce pita pockets into quarters; split each apart. Place wedges on prepared baking sheet. Bake 10 minutes, or until well toasted. Cool. Crackers can be stored in an airtight container.

Sauces and Toppings

Berry Syrup

Yields: 8 servings
1 serving (1 tablespoon):
Calories   = 20   *Exchanges = ½ Fruit*
Cholesterol = 0 mg
Fat   = 0 gm
Sodium   = 0 mg

2 cups berries (blueberries, strawberries, raspberries)
2 tablespoons pineapple juice concentrate
½ teaspoon vanilla

Blend berries in a food processor. Combine all ingredients
in a heavy saucepan. Bring to a boil and simmer for 25 to
30 minutes. Cool before serving.

Italian Tomato Sauce

Yields: 14 servings
1 serving (½ cup):
Calories   = 40   *Exchanges = 1½ Vegetable*
Cholesterol = 0 mg
Fat   = 0 gm
Sodium   = 150 mg

2 large cans (28-ounce each) crushed Italian tomatoes
1 teaspoon dried basil
½ teaspoon dried oregano
*1 6-ounce can tomato paste
1 bay leaf
10 minced garlic cloves
½ teaspoon pepper

Mix all ingredients and simmer on stove for 2 hours. Use for lasagna, stuffed shells, or any other recipe you desire.

Lower-Sodium Variation:
  Substitute low-sodium tomato paste.
  1 serving: Sodium = 20 mg

Original Tomato Sauce

Yields: 6 servings
1 serving (¾ cup):

Calories = 100	Exchanges = 2½ Vegetable +
Cholesterol = 0 mg	½ Fat
Fat = 3 gm	
Sodium = 10 mg	

  ½ to 1 minced garlic clove
  1 tablespoon olive oil
  4 pounds fresh Italian tomatoes
  1 small chopped onion
  ½ chopped pablano pepper, seeded
  ½ teaspoon "lite" salt
  ½ chopped green pepper (optional)
    tabasco sauce (optional)

Lightly brown garlic in olive oil. Cut tomatoes in small chunks. Add tomatoes to garlic along with onion, pablano pepper, salt, and green pepper, if used. Cook on high until tomatoes soften; then lower heat and cook 20 minutes. Add tabasco sauce to taste, if desired. Use as desired.

Spicy Tomato Sauce

Yields: 8 servings
1 serving (4 tablespoons):
Calories   = 28   *Exchanges = 1 Vegetable*
Cholesterol = 0 mg
Fat   = 0 gm
Sodium   = 340 mg

    2 8-ounce cans low-sodium tomato sauce
    1 4-ounce can chopped green chiles, undrained
    1 minced garlic clove
 ¾ cup chopped green onion
    2 teaspoons chili powder
    1 teaspoon ground cumin
 ¼ teaspoon dried whole oregano

Combine all ingredients in saucepan; simmer, uncovered,
for 5 minutes.

5

Watch the Way You Respond— and Learn to Relax!

Practically everyone has anxious, worried, or otherwise tense reactions to highly stressful situations. But *not* everyone experiences a significant rise in blood pressure as a result of stress.

The blood pressure in some people rises only slightly, if at all, under extreme emotional pressure—though there will typically be a marked increase in the heart rate. Others experience a moderate rise in pressure, perhaps into the mild hypertensive range just above 140/90 mm Hg. Still others—who are called "vascular reactors"—undergo a major "spike" in their measurements, well up into the moderate or even severe range, in excess of 200/110.

There is evidence, as we saw in chapter 3 on risk factors related to hypertension, that people who are under constant stress are more likely to develop sustained hypertension than are those in tranquil environments. Furthermore, this risk seems greatest among the vascular reactors—those whose blood pressure increases rapidly under stress.

The periodic expansion of the vessels through temporarily high readings finally takes its toll: The muscles in the vessel walls thicken, and the tissue on the inner lining of the vessel walls becomes scarred and vulnerable to the buildup of fatty or atherosclerotic deposits. The end result of these and other influences is an increase in the resistance of the vessels to the pressure of the flowing blood—and permanent hypertension.

In many cases, this reactor response to stress is probably related to genetic factors. It's been suggested, for example, that some people inherit a sympathetic nervous system that responds more sensitively to stress than is the case with other people. Also, genetic problems in the sodium excretion mechanism may contribute to higher blood pressure readings.

A 1983 study of young men with normal blood pressure was reported in *Science* by researcher K. C. Light and several colleagues. A major finding: Stress can trigger disturbances in the sodium excretion mechanism in the children of hypertensives.

Specifically, in a majority of the young male participants with hypertensive parents, one hour of emotional stress caused a fall in their sodium excretion. Such a decline in sodium loss will automatically encourage greater sodium retention in the blood, a higher blood volume—and a concomitant rise in blood pressure.

But among the participants whose parents had *normal* blood pressure, sodium excretion actually *increased* with stress—a result that tends to decrease blood volume and be protective against the development of hypertension.

Finally, those with the lower excretion levels of sodium during the stressful hour tended also to have the greatest increases in heart rate under stress. This response was important because, as we know, another major factor in regulating blood pressure is the pumping action of the heart.

To summarize: The elevated blood pressure in the participants in this study occurred as a result of (1) the increase in blood volume due to excess sodium retention, and (2) the increase in the heart rate. Furthermore, both the sodium excretion deficiency *and* the greater rise in heart rate during stress seem to be inherited or genetically related.

However, this doesn't mean that a person who has

inherited some undesirable traits must be destined to a life of hypertension. On the contrary, there are a number of effective ways to combat the impact of stress, which I've classified under two general headings: (1) relaxation techniques, and (2) lifestyle habits.

Combating Stress Through Relaxation Techniques

A number of studies have shown that various relaxation techniques—including various forms of meditation, biofeedback programs, and muscle-relaxing strategies—can help lower both diastolic and systolic readings, at least temporarily.

For example, in a 1981 study reported in the *British Medical Journal*, medical researcher Chandra Patel and two colleagues found that eight weeks of relaxation therapy, reinforced by biofeedback techniques, could lower average systolic pressure from more than 160 mm Hg to 142 mm Hg, and diastolic readings from 100 mm Hg to less than 90 mm Hg.

In a later investigation in 1988 in the *British Medical Journal*, using similar relaxation and biofeedback approaches, Patel and Michael Marmot reported similar results: After one year of treatment, average systolic pressure dropped more than 12 mm Hg lower for those on relaxation treatment, in comparison with a control group not on such treatment. Also, diastolic pressures dropped more than 4 mm Hg on average for those on relaxation therapy.

Generally speaking, relaxation therapy is also helpful when used with antihypertensive medications. A study by Dr. Rolf G. Jacob and five colleagues, published in the *Archives of Internal Medicine* in 1986, explored the effect of using relaxation techniques with a beta blocker (100 mg per day of atenolol) and also with a diuretic (50 mg per day of chlorthalidone).

The researchers concluded that the long-term effects

of relaxation were beneficial, independent of the medication therapy. At the same time, although relaxation enhanced the action of both drugs, it worked best with the diuretic in lowering blood pressure.

Why did the diuretic, combined with relaxation, work best? The researchers suggest that relaxation therapy may somehow enhance the effect of diuretic drugs on the kidneys and sympathetic nervous system. But they indicate that further exploration of the biological mechanisms is necessary before any definite explanation can be offered.

A number of hypertension experts have concluded that for the average patient, the impact of relaxation therapy is "modest." Also, they note that the benefits often are limited, lasting for only a short time.

On the other hand, some highly motivated patients find that they can achieve significant, lasting drops in their blood pressure with regular relaxation therapy. These people have discovered that relaxation therapy can play a key role in controlling hypertensive conditions *without* drugs.

In general, I recommend a systematic relaxation technique for anyone who has hypertension. It's not uncommon for those who are diligent with this approach to see drops of 10 mm Hg or more in both their diastolic and systolic readings.

If you decide to try relaxation therapy, what approach should you use? Some of the techniques, such as those using sophisticated biofeedback machines, are too expensive and complicated for the average patient. But the following method—based on several concepts, including the classic "relaxation response" approach popularized by Dr. Herbert Benson of Harvard Medical School—is easy to use and produces beneficial results in many people:

- Find a quiet room or corner; sit comfortably, with your back straight, feet flat on the floor, and eyes closed. Your arms should rest loosely and comfortably in your lap.

- For about one minute, concentrate on relaxing all the muscles in your body. Begin by tensing and then relaxing your feet and legs, your trunk muscles, your neck and shoulder muscles, and your arms and hands.

- For another ten minutes, breathe regularly. Every time you exhale, repeat silently a particular word or phrase that makes you feel comfortable or secure. Many people choose a meaningful word or two from their religious faith.

- When outside thoughts threaten to interrupt this relaxation exercise—as they always will—don't fight them. Simply push them gently aside and return to your "focus word," as Dr. Benson calls it.

- Include one or two of these relaxation therapy sessions in your schedule each day, and you might be surprised to discover what happens to your blood pressure.

- Another possibility is what Dr. Benson calls a "mini-meditation." That is, in addition to your lengthier relaxation sessions, try doing your regular breathing with your focus word or phrase for much shorter periods—even a few seconds, if that's all the time you have.

As I've said, this approach doesn't work for everyone, and it may not work for you. However, it *has* succeeded quite well in helping control hypertension in many people, and it *may* work for you. So why not try it?

You may find that these relaxation sessions become the cornerstone to the next approach to stress management—combating the pressures in your life through certain lifestyle strategies.

Combating Stress Through Creative Lifestyle Strategies

The first way to control your response to stress is to develop a basic relaxation technique, such as the one described in the preceding section. Next, it's important to learn to apply shortened forms of that technique and also other, simple relaxation devices, such as taking a deep breath, during your most stressful times.

Here's an easy-to-use daily stress management strategy, based on those employed by Chandra Patel and other investigators in their research on relaxation therapy and hypertension:

Step 1. Identify those times of day when you're under the greatest stress. You probably already know when your anxiety levels are most likely to rise and when feelings of being out of control are most likely to occur.

Even better, if you have a home blood pressure device, use it to determine those times during a typical day when your blood pressure peaks. If possible, take your blood pressure before, after, or even during your high-pressure situations. (Obviously, you can't strap a cuff around your upper arm during a business meeting. But you may be able to take your pressure during a phone conversation in the privacy of your office.)

By evaluating your feelings or actually determining your blood pressure, you'll be in a better position to answer these questions:

- Are you under the greatest stress when you're on the telephone, trying to negotiate a business deal or make a sale?

- How about the encounters you have with your boss, or presentations you are required to make to committees or colleagues?

- Do your worst on-the-job experiences involve conducting interviews with strangers? Getting your office organized in preparation for a trip? Making the transition back into the office after you've been away for a few days?

Researchers have found that for many people, the most stressful times occur when they are *outside* the office—such as driving to and from work; waiting for red lights to change; dealing with air or rail travel; or waiting for a dental appointment. Some find that they experience the most stress in encounters with their spouse or children, or even at church or synagogue meetings.

Whatever your worst times for stress, write down the precise situations and the hours of the day when they most often occur. This way, they won't catch you by surprise, and you'll be in a better position to prepare for them and meet them with greater equanimity.

Step 2. Formulate a response strategy to meet these difficult situations.

An approach that has helped many hypertensives is to employ a brief relaxation technique (e.g., a "mini-meditation") just before and after the event. So, if you're expecting a particularly difficult phone conversation, take a minute or so beforehand to relax your muscles; concentrate on your breathing; and silently repeat your focus word or phrase. Then, proceed with the conversation. Finally, *immediately* after you hang up, employ the relaxation technique again for a minute or so.

If you can discipline yourself to follow this strategy, you'll likely be pleased with the results. Many people find that they feel calmer, are able to handle themselves more effectively during stressful encounters, and blood pressure readings taken on home devices reveal that their measurements are lower.

Step 3. Condition yourself to engage in relaxation techniques *during* stressful situations that you may not be able to anticipate.

Many times, high-pressure encounters are impossible to foresee. In those circumstances—and even when you *are* able to anticipate a source of stress—you may find it helpful to close your eyes for a second or two and concentrate on regular breathing and on silently repeating your focus word. In fact, just a deep breath or two may be enough to calm you down and reduce your stress level.

Step 4. Learn to *detach* yourself from the stress in your life.

For example, if you begin to get into an argument with a business associate, you might imagine yourself in another office, or in an airplane flying over the city, or even on a quiet tropical beach.

It also may be helpful to say to yourself, "This isn't that important. It's silly for me to get so excited about a little problem that's bound to pass."

Achieving detachment will enable you to put the pressure you're feeling in proper perspective. In fact, when you think about it, *almost nothing* that we do in our daily lives is so important that it justifies our getting excessively anxious, angry, or tense.

Certainly, some level of anger or anxiety is inevitable for busy, ambitious, high-achieving people. But when these emotions paralyze, immobilize, or upset a person to any extent, the emotional and physical fallout may be unacceptable. The patient will most likely find that it's impossible to function effectively—and blood pressure levels are much more likely to increase.

So, learning to watch the way you respond to stress is a very personal endeavor. Some people have the ability and discipline to develop a relaxation strategy, and others don't. A few may find that no relaxation technique helps. But *most* should discover that a systematic approach to relaxation is a valuable tool in controlling hypertension.

The ultimate question is simply this: How willing are you to make a commitment to use a regular relaxation technique—and to make some significant adjustments in your lifestyle? Such commitments and adjustments are required to minimize the impact of stress in your life. And don't forget what I've said many times previously: Aerobic exercise performed regularly is nature's best physiological tranquilizer.

6

A Future Without Hypertension?

Because of the effective work of many physicians and other health professionals, as well as the National High Blood Pressure Program—an effort by the National Heart, Lung and Blood Institute, which was launched in 1972—a great deal of progress has been made in recent years in combating the ravages of hypertension.

The public has been given access to free blood pressure measurements in shopping malls and on street corners; literature showing how to lower the risks of hypertension has been disseminated on a large scale; and physicians have been alerted as never before to the gravity of the problem.

The results of this public-information campaign have been dramatic. Since 1972, there has been a 50 percent decline in the national age-adjusted stroke mortality rate (stroke, as you know, is one of the major lethal complications of hypertension). Also, the death rate from coronary artery disease has declined by 35 percent during that period.

But much more needs to be done. There are currently *at least* 40 million adult Americans whose average blood pressure exceeds 140/90 mm Hg. By definition, these people are hypertensives, and their disease *could* eventually place them at serious risk to their health or their lives.

Fortunately, a growing percentage of these hypertensives—a majority, by most estimates—are on appropriate drugs or under regular medical care. Increasing numbers of those who have high blood pressure, or are at significant risk for the disease, are watching their diets, exercising, trying to manage stress more effectively, and seeing their physicians regularly.

Still, I continue to be profoundly concerned about getting the word out to those who, for whatever reason, aren't aware of the danger they face. I'm also deeply disturbed by those who may be aware but have failed to take decisive action against hypertension.

I frequently encounter patients who tell me, in effect, "I know I have a *little* hypertension, but it's not *that* bad. Besides, I know it takes years for complications to develop." Or, "I simply don't have the discipline to stay on an exercise program." Or, "My schedule just doesn't allow for a serious commitment to a low-salt diet." Or, "I keep forgetting to take my blood pressure medication."

How do you motivate such patients? It's frustrating for doctors to diagnose the problem or identify multiple risk factors in a patient during an exam, and to communicate that danger clearly, and then have that patient disregard all your medical advice.

I don't believe in using scare tactics, though certainly there *is* reason for a patient to be deeply concerned if a set of blood pressure measurements reveals a high level of risk. But the main motivator, in my estimation, should be the promise of good future health and an enhanced quality of life.

If you have normal blood pressure, but you know you're at risk, why not act *now* through nondrug measures to lower your risk? Why wait and possibly have to go on medications or, worse, suffer a stroke or kidney damage?

If you have mild hypertension, why not be diligent *now* in following your physician's advice about changing your diet, exercise habits, and response to stress?

If you have more serious hypertension, why not be conscientious *now* about staying on your prescribed medication and *also* pursuing nondrug approaches to treatment? If you do, you may be able to reduce your drug dosage and perhaps even go off the medication completely at some point.

Likely, there will never be a future entirely without hypertension. But if we get more serious about making the best use of the medical tools at hand—and they are powerful tools, indeed—most people should eventually find that high blood pressure is a condition that *should* and *can* be brought completely under control.

R

References

Chapter 1

Kaplan, Norman M., M.D. *Clinical Hypertension*. Baltimore: Williams & Wilkins, fourth edition, 1986.

————. *Management of Hypertension*. Durant, Oklahoma: Creative Infomatics, Inc., second edition, 1987.

"The 1988 Report of the Joint National Committee on Detection, Evaluation, and Treatment of High Blood Pressure." *Archives of Internal Medicine,* vol. 148, May 1988, pp. 1023–37.

Chapter 2

"Blood-Pressure Monitors." *Consumer Reports,* May 1987, pp. 314–19.

Evans, C. Edward, et al. "Home Blood Pressure Measuring Devices: A Comparative Study of Accuracy." *Journal of Hypertension,* vol. 7, 1989, pp. 133–42.

Hampton, J. R. "Mild Hypertension: To Treat or Not to Treat?" *Comparative Studies in Hypertension.* Nephron 47: suppl. 1, pp. 57–61 (1987).

Hunt, James C., et al. "Devices Used for Self-Measurement of Blood Pressure." *Archives of Internal Medicine,* vol. 145, December 1985, pp. 2231–34.

Kaplan, Norman M., M.D. *Clinical Hypertension.* Baltimore: Williams & Wilkins, fourth edition, 1986.

———. *Management of Hypertension.* Durant, Oklahoma: Creative Infomatics, Inc., second edition, 1987.

———. "Misdiagnosis of Systemic Hypertension and Recommendations for Improvement." *American Journal of Cardiology,* vol. 60, December 1, 1987, pp. 1383–86.

"The 1988 Report of the Joint National Committee on Detection, Evaluation, and Treatment of High Blood Pressure." *Archives of Internal Medicine,* vol. 148, May 1988, pp. 1023–37.

Pickering, Thomas G., et al. "How Common Is White Coat Hypertension?" *Journal of the American Medical Association,* vol. 259, no. 2, January 8, 1988, pp. 225–28.

Chapter 3

Arakawa, Kikuo, et al. "The Beneficial Effect of Exercise Therapy for Essential Hypertension and a Probable Mechanism: A Preliminary Report." *Nutritional Prevention of Cardiovascular Disease,* 1984, pp. 349–55.

"Diuretics, Hypokalemia, and Ventricular Ectopy: The Controversy Continues." *Archives of Internal Medicine,* vol. 145, July 1985, pp. 1185–87.

Duncan, John J., et al. "The Effects of Aerobic Exercise on Plasma Catecholamines and Blood Pressure in Patients with Mild Essential Hypertension." *Journal of the American Medical Association,* vol. 254, no. 18, November 8, 1985, pp. 2609–13.

el-Dean, Salah, M.D., et al. "Physical Exercise and Health: A Review Study." *Medical Times,* vol. 113, no. 12, December 1985, pp. 57–64.

"Hypertension." 1988 Consensus Conference on Exercise, Fitness and Health, held in Toronto, Canada, section D, paragraph 309.

Jingu, Sumie, M.D., et al. "Exercise Training Augments Cardiopulmonary Baroreflex Control of Forearm Vascular Resistance in Middle-Aged Subjects." *Japanese Circulation Journal,* vol. 52, February 1988.

Kaplan, Norman M., M.D. "Calcium and Potassium in the Treatment of Essential Hypertension." *Seminars in Nephrology,* vol. 8, no. 2, June 1988, pp. 176–84.

———. *Clinical Hypertension.* Baltimore: Williams & Wilkins, fourth edition, 1986.

———. *Management of Hypertension.* Durant, Oklahoma: Creative Infomatics, Inc., second edition, 1987.

———. "Non-Drug Treatment of Hypertension." *Annals of Internal Medicine,* vol. 102, no. 3, March 1985, pp. 359–73.

Khaw, Kay-Tee, and Elizabeth Barrett-Connor. "Dietary Fiber and Reduced Ischemic Heart Disease Mortality Rates in Men and Women: A 12-year Prospective Study." *American Journal of Epidemiology,* vol. 126, no. 6, 1987, pp. 1093–1102.

Kiyonaga, Akira, et al. "Blood Pressure and Hormonal Responses to Aerobic Exercise." *Hypertension,* vol. 7, no. 1, January–February 1985, pp. 125–31.

Larson, Eric B., and Robert A. Bruce. "Health Benefits of Exercise in an Aging Society." *Archives of Internal Medicine,* vol. 147, February 1987, pp. 353–56.

Liao, Youlian, et al. "Cardiovascular Responses to Exercise of Participants in a Trial on the Primary Prevention of Hypertension." *Journal of Hypertension,* vol. 5, no. 3, 1987, pp. 317–21.

McNutt, Robert A., M.D., et al. "Acute Myocardial Infarction in a 22-year-old World Class Weight Lifter Using Anabolic Steroids." *American Journal of Cardiology,* vol. 62, July 1, 1988, p. 164.

"The 1988 Report of the Joint National Committee on Detection, Evaluation, and Treatment of High Blood

Pressure." *Archives of Internal Medicine,* vol. 148, May 1988, pp. 1023–37.

Ravussin, Eric, Ph.D., et al. "Reduced Rate of Energy Expenditure as a Risk Factor for Body-Weight Gain." *New England Journal of Medicine,* vol. 318, no. 8, February 25, 1988, pp. 467–72.

Slattery, Martha L. and David R. Jacobs, Jr. "Physical Fitness and Cardiovascular Disease Mortality: The U.S. Railroad Study." *American Journal of Epidemiology,* vol. 127, no. 3, 1988, pp. 571–80.

Urata, Hidenori, et al. "Antihypertensive and Volume-Depleting Effects of Mild Exercise on Essential Hypertension." *Hypertension,* vol. 9, no. 3, March 1987, pp. 245–52.

Chapter 4

Altura, Burton M., and Bella T. Altura. "Interactions of Mg and K on Blood Vessels—Aspects in View of Hypertension. Review of Present Status and New Findings." *Magnesium,* vol. 3, 1984, pp. 175–94.

Beilin, Lawrence J. "State of the Art Lecture, Diet and Hypertension: Critical Concepts and Controversies." *Journal of Hypertension,* vol. 5, suppl. 5, 1987, pp. S447–57.

"Calcium and Hypertension." *Nutrition and the M.D.,* July 1985.

Fregley, Melvin J. "Estimates of Sodium and Potassium Intake." *Annals of Internal Medicine,* vol. 98, May 1983, pp. 792–99.

Kaplan, Norman M., M.D. *Clinical Hypertension.* Baltimore: Williams & Wilkins, fourth edition, 1986.

———. *Management of Hypertension.* Durant, Oklahoma: Creative Infomatics, Inc., second edition, 1987.

Kostas, G. and K. Glasgow. "Limit Your Sodium!" *The Balancing Act.* Dallas: 1984.

Kroenke, Kurt, et al. "The Value of Serum Magnesium

Determination in Hypertensive Patients Receiving Diuretics." *Archives of Internal Medicine,* vol. 147, September 1987, pp. 1553–56.

"Magnesium Aspartate and 'Jogger's Heart.'" *Health News,* May–July 1982.

"The 1988 Report of the Joint National Committee on Detection, Evaluation, and Treatment of High Blood Pressure." *Archives of Internal Medicine,* vol. 148, May 1988, pp. 1023–37.

Resnick, Lawrence M. "Dietary Calcium and Hypertension." *Journal of Nutrition,* vol. 117, 1987, pp. 1806–08.

Siani, Alfonso, et al. "Controlled Trial of Long-Term Oral Potassium Supplements in Patients with Mild Hypertension." *British Medical Journal,* vol. 294, June 6, 1987, pp. 1453–56.

Solum, T. T., et al. "The Influence of a High-Fibre Diet on Body Weight, Serum Lipids, and Blood Pressure in Slightly Overweight Persons." *International Journal of Obesity,* vol. 11, suppl. 1, 1987, pp. 67–71.

Stamier, Rose, M.A., et al. "Nutritional Therapy for High Blood Pressure, Final Report of a Four-Year Randomized Controlled Trial—The Hypertension Control Program." *Journal of the American Medical Association,* vol. 257, no. 11, March 20, 1987, pp. 1484–91.

Weinberger, Myron H., M.D. "Salt Intake and Blood Pressure in Humans." *Contemporary Nutrition,* vol. 13, no. 8, 1988.

Williams, Paul T., Ph.D., et al. "Associations of Dietary Fat, Regional Adiposity, and Blood Pressure in Men." *Journal of the American Medical Association,* vol. 257, no. 23, June 19, 1987, pp. 3251–56.

Chapter 5

Benson, Herbert, M.D. *Beyond the Relaxation Response.* New York: Berkley, 1984.

————. *The Relaxation Response*. New York: Avon, 1976.

————. *Your Maximum Mind*. New York: Avon, 1987.

Ewart, Craig K., et al. "Feasibility and Effectiveness of School-Based Relaxation in Lowering Blood Pressure." *Health Psychology*, vol. 6, 1987, pp. 399–416.

Goleman, Daniel. "Hypertension? Relax." *New York Times Magazine*, December 11, 1988.

Jacob, Rolf G., et al. "The Behavioral Treatment of Hypertension: Long-Term Effects." *Behavior Therapy*, vol. 18, 1987, pp. 325–52.

————. "Relaxation Therapy for Hypertension: Comparison of Effects with Concomitant Placebo, Diuretic, and B-Blocker." *Archives of Internal Medicine*, vol. 146, December 1986, pp. 2335–40.

Kaplan, Norman M., M.D. *Clinical Hypertension*. Baltimore: Williams & Wilkins, fourth edition, 1986.

————. *Management of Hypertension*. Durant, Oklahoma: Creative Infomatics, Inc., second edition, 1987.

"The 1988 Report of the Joint National Committee on Detection, Evaluation, and Treatment of High Blood Pressure." *Archives of Internal Medicine*, vol. 148, May 1988, pp. 1023–37.

Patel, Chandra, and Michael Marmot. "Can General Practitioners Use Training in Relaxation and Management of Stress to Reduce Mild Hypertension?" *British Medical Journal*, vol. 296, January 2, 1988, pp. 21–24.

Warner, Greg. "Blood Pressure Was 'Up.'" *Baptist Standard*, November 17, 1982.

Chapter 6

"The 1988 Report of the Joint National Committee on Detection, Evaluation, and Treatment of High Blood Pressure." *Archives of Internal Medicine*, vol. 148, May 1988, pp. 1023–37.

I

Sodium, Potassium, Calcium, and Fiber Content of Selected Foods

Sodium

0– 140 mg Sodium	141–400 mg Sodium	401 + mg Sodium

FRUIT and VEGETABLE
(½ cup or 1 small serving)

0– 140 mg Sodium	141–400 mg Sodium	401 + mg Sodium
Fruit, fresh or frozen or canned— 1–50 mg	Beets, canned— 200 mg	Pork and beans, canned—590 mg
Frozen lima beans— 125 mg	Cream-style corn— 300 mg	Sauerkraut, canned—880 mg
Frozen peas— 90 mg	Tomato juice— 243 mg	Spaghetti sauce— 925 mg
Tomato paste— 50 mg		Tomato sauce— 656 mg
Vegetables, canned—300 mg		Vegetable soup, canned—505 mg
Vegetables, plain, frozen— 10–30 mg		

BREAD/STARCH (½ cup or 1 piece)

0– 140 mg Sodium	141–400 mg Sodium
Graham crackers— 95 mg	Biscuit—270 mg
Noodles—2 mg	Bran flakes— 182 mg
Rice—2 mg	Corn flakes— 163 mg
Saltine crackers (4)—125 mg	Cornbread—265 mg
Shredded Wheat— 1 mg	Cream of wheat— 175 mg
Wheat bread— 130 mg	Instant oatmeal— 350 mg
	Waffle—340 mg
	Wheaties—158 mg

0–140 mg Sodium	141–400 mg Sodium	401 + mg Sodium

MILK
(8 ounces milk or yogurt or 1 ounce cheese)

0–140 mg Sodium	141–400 mg Sodium	401 + mg Sodium
Low-fat yogurt, fruit—120 mg	Buttermilk—318 mg	American processed cheese—405 mg
Low-sodium cheese—90 mg	Cheddar cheese— 175 mg	Low-fat cottage cheese (½ cup)— 455 mg
Mozzarella cheese— 104 mg	Chocolate milk— 150 mg	
Skim milk—125 mg	Chocolate pudding— 320 mg	
Swiss cheese— 75 mg	Low-fat milk, 2%— 145 mg	
Whole milk— 120 mg	Low-fat yogurt, plain—159 mg	

MEAT (3 ounces or as specified)

0–140 mg Sodium	141–400 mg Sodium	401 + mg Sodium
Beef—52 mg	Beef liver—155 mg	Baked ham— 800 mg
Chicken—74 mg	Peanut butter (2 tablespoons)— 190 mg	Bologna—1036 mg
Egg (1)—60 mg		Corned beef— 808 mg
Pork chop—54 mg		Frankfurter (1)— 477 mg
		Sausage—788 mg
		Tuna—727 mg

0–140 mg Sodium	141–400 mg Sodium	401 + mg Sodium

COMBINATION FOODS

0–140 mg Sodium	141–400 mg Sodium	401 + mg Sodium
Fresh fruit salad (1 cup)—10 mg Tossed salad (1 cup) with oil and vinegar (1 tablespoon)—12 mg	Homemade soup (1 cup)—400 mg	Chicken noodle soup, canned (1 cup)—1999 mg Beef stew, canned (1 cup)—980 mg Spaghetti and meatballs, canned (1½ cup)—985 mg Chicken pot pie (1)—863 mg Chili with beans and beef (1 cup)—1355 mg Chow mein (1 cup)—725 mg Fast food fish sandwich—800 mg Fast food hamburger—774 mg Frozen beef dinner—938 mg Pizza with sausage (1 slice)—720 mg

OTHER FOODS
(½ cup or 1 piece or as specified)

0–140 mg Sodium	141–400 mg Sodium	401 + mg Sodium
Beer—8 mg Coffee—2 mg Cola—2 mg Ice cream—90 mg Oatmeal cookie—69 mg Sherbet—20 mg Wine—5 mg	Cake-type doughnut—216 mg Potato chips (10)—200 mg Salted popcorn—233 mg Sweet pickle—200 mg	Apple pie—482 mg Dill pickle—1930 mg

0–140 mg Sodium	141–400 mg Sodium	401 + mg Sodium

FATS and CONDIMENTS
(1 tablespoon or as specified)

0–140 mg Sodium	141–400 mg Sodium	401 + mg Sodium
Barbecue sauce—130 mg	Bacon (3 slices)—303 mg	Baking powder (1 teaspoon)—405 mg
Butter—120 mg	Catsup—155 mg	Baking soda (1 teaspoon)—821 mg
Cooking wine—133 mg	French dressing—220 mg	Bouillon cube (1 teaspoon)—960 mg
Herbs and spices (1 teaspoon)—1 mg	Horseradish—165 mg	Garlic salt (1 teaspoon)—1850 mg
Margarine—150 mg	Italian dressing—315 mg	Green olives (5)—465 mg
Margarine, unsalted—0 mg	Low-sodium soy sauce—300 mg	Lite salt (1 teaspoon)—1100 mg
Mayonnaise—85 mg	Worcestershire sauce—157 mg	Meat tenderizer (1 teaspoon)—1750 mg
Oil—0 mg		Monosodium glutamate (MSG) (1 teaspoon)—492 mg
Parsley—12 mg		Onion salt (1 teaspoon)—1590 mg
Picante sauce—74 mg		Soy sauce—1332 mg
Prepared mustard—65 mg		Table salt (1 teaspoon)—2132 mg
Salt substitute—0 mg		
Tartar sauce—50 mg		

Potassium

401 + mg Potassium	200–400 mg Potassium	0–199 mg Potassium

MILK
(8 ounces milk or yogurt or 1 ounce cheese)

401 + mg Potassium	200–400 mg Potassium	0–199 mg Potassium
Chocolate milk— 417 mg	Buttermilk—342 mg	American cheese— 45 mg
Low-fat milk— 450 mg	Skim milk—381 mg	Cheddar cheese— 30 mg
Low-fat yogurt, plain—530 mg	Whole milk—370 mg	Chocolate pudding— 170 mg
	Yogurt, fruit— 400 mg	Cottage cheese— 95 mg
		Swiss cheese— 30 mg

FRUIT and VEGETABLE
(½ cup or 1 small serving)

401 + mg Potassium	200–400 mg Potassium	0–199 mg Potassium
Baked potato— 780 mg	Broccoli—205 mg	Apple juice—125 mg
Banana—440 mg	Carrots, raw— 245 mg	Apple sauce—100 mg
Cantaloupe—401 mg	Mashed potato— 260 mg	Collard greens— 170 mg
Figs (2)—640 mg	Nectarine—294 mg	Fruit cocktail—25 mg
Prunes—528 mg	Orange juice— 370 mg	Green beans—95 mg
		Pear, canned— 130 mg

BREAD/STARCH (½ cup or 1 piece)

401 + mg Potassium	200–400 mg Potassium	0–199 mg Potassium
Bran Buds—700 mg	Bran flakes—248 mg	Corn flakes—24 mg
Wheat bran (1 tablespoon)— 460 mg	Bran Chex—228 mg	Farina—10 mg
	Kidney beans— 335 mg	Graham cracker— 55 mg
	Lentils—250 mg	Noodles—45 mg
	Navy beans—360 mg	Oatmeal—75 mg
		Rice—40 mg
		Saltines (4)—15 mg
		Wheat bread—70 mg
		White bread—25 mg

401 + mg Potassium	200–400 mg Potassium	0–199 mg Potassium

MEAT (3 ounces or as specified)

401 + mg Potassium	200–400 mg Potassium	0–199 mg Potassium
Cod—420 mg	Beef liver—325 mg	Bacon (3 slices)—92 mg
Scallops—455 mg	Chicken—243 mg	Beef—185 mg
Sole—585 mg	Ham, canned—304 mg	Bologna (1 ounce)—65 mg
	Pork chop—287 mg	Egg (1)—65 mg
	Tuna fish—275 mg	Frankfurter (1)—95 mg
	Turkey—350 mg	Peanut butter (1 tablespoon)—100 mg
		Sausage (1 ounce)—105 mg
		Shrimp—105 mg

COMBINATION FOODS

401 + mg Potassium	200–400 mg Potassium	0–199 mg Potassium
Beef stew, canned (1 cup)—615 mg	Fast food fish sandwich—250 mg	Chicken noodle soup, canned (1 cup)—55 mg
Burrito, bean and cheese (1)—479 mg	Spaghetti with meatballs, canned (1 cup)—355 mg	Chicken pot pie (1)—172 mg
Chow mein (1 cup)—420 mg	Stuffed pepper (1)—270 mg	Pizza with sausage (1 slice)—160 mg
Fast food hamburger, jumbo—454 mg		
Frozen beef dinner—655 mg		
Lasagna (1 cup)—740 mg		
Spaghetti with meat sauce (1 cup)—592 mg		

401 + mg Potassium	200–400 mg Potassium	0–199 mg Potassium

OTHER FOODS
(1 cup or 1 piece or as specified)

Avocado (½)—
680 mg

Banana pudding
(½ cup)—403 mg

Ice cream (1 cup)—
520 mg

Postum
(1 teaspoon)—
896 mg

Danish pastry—
275 mg

Dill pickle—270 mg

Peanuts
(2 tablespoons)—
200 mg

Potato chips (10)—
225 mg

Beer (12 ounces)—
90 mg

Butter
(1 teaspoon)—
1 mg

Coffee—80 mg

Cola (12 ounces)—
trace

Margarine
(1 teaspoon)—
1 mg

Oatmeal cookie—
20 mg

Orange sherbet—
21 mg

Pretzels (1 cup)—
39 mg

Vanilla ice cream—
130 mg

Vanilla wafers (3)—
51 mg

Wine (4 ounces)—
95 mg

CONDIMENTS (1 tablespoon or as specified)

Black strap
molasses—
585 mg

Tomato sauce
(½ cup)—463 mg

Parsley—219 mg

Italian dressing—
2 mg

Mayonnaise—15 mg

Oregano—99 mg

Paprika—147 mg

Pepper—75 mg

Prepared mustard—
15 mg

Sage—33 mg

Thyme—150 mg

Calcium

270 + mg Calcium	150–269 mg Calcium	80–149 mg Calcium

MILK
(8 ounces milk or yogurt or 1 ounce cheese)

Buttermilk—285 mg	American cheese—175 mg	
Chocolate milk—285 mg	Blue cheese—150 mg	
Skim milk—300 mg	Brick cheese—204 mg	
Low-fat milk, 1%—300 mg	Cheddar cheese—204 mg	
Low-fat milk, 2%—300 mg	Colby cheese—195 mg	
Whole milk—290 mg	Edam cheese—207 mg	
Low-fat yogurt, fruit—345 mg	Monterey cheese—212 mg	
Low-fat yogurt, plain—415 mg	Mozzarella cheese, part-skim—180 mg	
Swiss cheese—270 mg	Mozzarella cheese—150 mg	
	Muenster cheese—203 mg	
	Ricotta cheese, part-skim (1 ounce = ¼ cup)—170 mg	

FRUIT and VEGETABLE
(½ cup or 1 small serving)

	Collards—180 mg	Bokchoy—125 mg
	Kale—150 mg	Mustard greens—100 mg
	Turnip greens—169 mg	

BREAD/STARCH (½ cup or 1 piece)

		Cornbread—135 mg
		Pancake—115 mg
		Waffle—130 mg

270 + mg Calcium	*150–269 mg Calcium*	*80–149 mg Calcium*

MEAT (3 ounces)

Sardines, with bones—370 mg	Salmon, with bones—170 mg	Beans dried, cooked—90 mg Oysters, raw—130 mg Tofu, processed with calcium sulfate—108 mg

COMBINATION FOODS

Macaroni and cheese (1 cup)—360 mg	Cream of mushroom soup with milk (1 cup)—178 mg Cream of tomato soup with milk (1 cup)—159 mg Taco, bean and cheese (1)—260 mg	Cheese pizza (1 piece)—145 mg Chili with beans (1 cup)—43 mg Spaghetti, meatballs, tomato sauce, and cheese (1 cup)—131 mg

OTHER FOODS (½ cup or as specified)

Chocolate milkshake—198 mg Vanilla milkshake—229 mg	Custard, baked—150 mg	Ice cream—90 mg Ice milk—140 mg Molasses, blackstrap (¼ cup)—135 mg Pudding, chocolate—133 mg

Note: To consume 1,000 mg of calcium daily, try to eat 2 to 3 foods daily from left column and 2 to 3 foods daily from center and right columns.

Fiber

5 + gm Fiber	2–4 gm Fiber	0–1 gm Fiber

FRUIT
(½ cup or 1 small serving or as specified)

5 + gm Fiber	2–4 gm Fiber	0–1 gm Fiber
Blackberries— 5.2 gm	Apple with peel (1)— 3.1 gm	Grapefruit (½)— .6 gm
Prunes, dried (5)— 7.8 gm	Apricots, dried (5)— 3.2 gm	Peach with skin— 1 gm
	Banana (1)—2 gm	Pineapple—1.2 gm
	Dried dates (5)— 4 gm	Raisins (2 table-spoons)—1.3 gm
	Orange (1)—2.6 gm	
	Pear with peel (1)— 4.4 gm	
	Raspberries—3.3 gm	

VEGETABLE (½ cup or 1 small serving)

5 + gm Fiber	2–4 gm Fiber	0–1 gm Fiber
	Broccoli, cooked— 3.2 gm	Asparagus, cooked— 1.3 gm
	Brussels sprouts, cooked—2.3 gm	Bean sprouts— 1.7 gm
	Cabbage, cooked— 3.3 gm	Cauliflower, cooked—1.5 gm
	Corn, cooked— 3.3 gm	Carrots, cooked— 1.3 gm
	Potato with skin, baked—3.8 gm	Celery (1 stalk)— .5 gm
	Sweet potato—3 gm	Green beans, cooked—1.2 gm
		Onion—.8 gm
		Spinach, cooked— 1.7 gm
		Tomato—1.1 gm

5 + gm Fiber	*2–4 gm Fiber*	*0–1 gm Fiber*

BREAD/STARCH (½ cup or 1 piece)

All-Bran—12 gm	Bran muffin—3 gm	Nutri-Grain—1.2 gm
All-Bran with Extra Fiber—13 gm	Whole wheat bread— 2.1 gm	Rye bread—1.2 gm
Bran Buds—12 gm	Bran Chex—3.4 gm	Whole wheat pasta— 1.3 gm
Fiber One—13 gm	Corn Bran—4 gm	
100% Bran—14 gm	40% Bran Flakes— 3.2 gm	
Wheat bran— 10.2 gm	Oat bran, cooked— 3.3 gm	
Kidney beans— 10 gm	Oatmeal, cooked— 2 gm	
Navy beans—6 gm	Raisin bran—2.7 gm	
	Shredded Wheat— 2.4 gm	
	Brown rice, cooked—2.4 gm	
	Lentils, cooked— 2.8 gm	
	Lima beans, cooked—3.6 gm	
	Peas, cooked— 3.2 gm	

COMBINATION FOODS
(serving size as specified)

Baked beans (½ cup)—7 gm	Bean soup (1 cup)— 4.5 gm
Lentil soup (1 cup)—7 gm	

MISCELLANEOUS FOODS
(½ cup or as specified)

Almonds—10.3 gm	Popcorn (3 cups)— 4.8 gm
Peanuts—6.7 gm	Walnuts—2.6 gm
Sunflower seeds— 5 gm	

II

Computer Analyses of Sample Menus and Recipes

1,200-Calorie Menus

Day	Calories	Protein gm	Fat gm	Carbo-hydrate gm	Choles-terol mg	Calcium mg	Sodium mg
			Week 1				
Monday	1202	71	34	153	116	854	770
Tuesday	1252	66	40	157	336	997	1220
Wednesday	1163	70	27	160	67	1152	2046
Thursday	1187	65	39	144	338	899	1588
Friday	1225	58	37	165	100	696	1662
Saturday	1218	73	34	155	135	1073	1361
Sunday	1177	75	29	154	103	661	1248
AVERAGE	**1203**	**68** 23%	**34** 25%	**155** 52%	**170**	**905**	**1414**
			Week 2				
Monday	1222	65	37	171	171	944	1655
Tuesday	1182	65	36	169	154	930	1771
Wednesday	1255	57	36	166	112	826	1056
Thursday	1253	62	30	174	77	751	979
Friday	1239	65	35	162	133	1061	1629
Saturday	1234	71	40	150	270	972	1470
Sunday	1258	69	27	186	95	909	1376
AVERAGE	**1234**	**65** 21%	**34** 25%	**168** 54%	**144**	**913**	**1419**

1,500-Calorie Menus

Day	Calories	Protein gm	Fat gm	Carbo-hydrate gm	Choles-terol mg	Calcium mg	Sodium mg
				Week 1			
Monday	1524	76	40	215	134	1007	839
Tuesday	1485	69	45	201	343	911	1491
Wednesday	1540	77	36	227	80	1239	2180
Thursday	1500	68	40	217	305	871	1882
Friday	1576	77	48	209	132	899	1980
Saturday	1496	79	44	196	146	1233	1456
Sunday	1556	93	32	224	112	942	1741
AVERAGE	**1525**	**77**	**41**	**213**	**179**	**1014**	**1653**
		20%	24%	56%			
				Week 2			
Monday	1508	80	38	224	132	1073	1799
Tuesday	1457	84	34	212	193	1129	1654
Wednesday	1502	75	47	190	141	1160	1495
Thursday	1530	88	36	207	99	1029	1395
Friday	1442	80	39	192	165	1110	1858
Saturday	1513	87	46	214	286	1011	1801
Sunday	1489	85	33	216	112	1078	1633
AVERAGE	**1491**	**82**	**39**	**207**	**161**	**1084**	**1662**
		21%	24%	55%			

2,200-Calorie Menus

Day	Calories	Protein gm	Fat gm	Carbo- hydrate gm	Choles- terol mg	Calcium mg	Sodium mg
				Week 1			
Monday	2134	106	54	306	189	1402	1304
Tuesday	2086	104	62	278	164	1295	2136
Wednesday	2132	125	60	273	279	1323	2261
Thursday	2226	124	50	320	146	1369	1779
Friday	2180	95	72	288	187	978	1926
Saturday	2261	113	77	279	163	1900	2118
Sunday	2122	105	46	322	124	868	2150
AVERAGE	**2163**	**110** 20%	**60** 25%	**295** 55%	**179**	**1305**	**1953**
				Week 2			
Monday	2240	124	71	299	238	1321	2439
Tuesday	2147	112	50	317	215	1184	2015
Wednesday	2243	101	71	303	204	1511	1932
Thursday	2193	116	68	323	142	919	2146
Friday	2224	123	56	285	278	1683	2480
Saturday	2142	93	64	320	347	1020	2417
Sunday	2248	123	58	311	195	1386	2397
AVERAGE	**2205**	**113** 20%	**62** 25%	**308** 55%	**231**	**1289**	**2260**

Recipe Analysis Per Serving

Recipes	Amount	Calories	Sodium (mg)	Exchanges
Apple Oat Crisp	1 cup	165	80	2 Fruit 1 Bread ½ Fat
Apple Waldorf Salad	½ cup	90	76	1 Fruit 1 Fat
Beef Broccoli Stir-Fry	¼ recipe	349	736	4 Meat 2 Vegetable ½ Fat
Low-Sodium Beef Broccoli Stir-Fry	¼ recipe	349	544	4 Meat 2 Vegetable ½ Fat
Berry Syrup	1 tablespoon	20	0	½ Fruit
Bran Muffins	1 muffin	127	200	1 Bread ½ Fruit 1 Fat
Cold Pasta Salad	1 cup	240	412	1½ Bread ½ Meat 2 Vegetable ½ Fat
Low-Sodium Cold Pasta Salad	1 cup	265	163	1½ Bread ½ Meat 3 Vegetable ½ Fat
French Toast Puff	1 slice	215	230	1 Meat ⅛ Milk 1 Bread ½ Fruit
Fruit Smoothy	1 cup	100	85	1½ Milk
Gazpacho	¾ cup	60	24	1½ Vegetable ½ Fat
Grilled Sesame Chicken Breasts	4 ounces	265	590	3½ Meat ½ Fruit 1 Fat ½ Bread
Herbed Garlic Fish Fillets	3 ounces	146	202	3 Meat
Italian Rice and Peas	½ cup	134	206	1½ Bread ½ Fat
Low-Sodium Italian Rice and Peas	½ cup	134	87	1½ Bread ½ Fat
Italian Tomato Sauce	½ cup	40	150	1½ Vegetable

Recipes	Amount	Calories	Sodium (mg)	Exchanges
Low-Sodium Italian Tomato Sauce	½ cup	40	20	1½ Vegetable
Long Grain and Wild Rice Chicken Salad	½ cup	260	250	1 Meat 1 Bread 1 Fat ½ Vegetable ½ Fruit
Minestrone Soup	1 cup	100	170	1 Bread 1 Vegetable
Low-Sodium Minestrone Soup	1 cup	100	57	1 Bread 1 Vegetable
Oat Bran Muffins	1 mini-muffin	66	60	½ Bread ½ Fruit ½ Fat
Oatmeal Pancakes	1 5-inch	98	199	1 Bread ⅙ Milk
Original Tomato Sauce	¾ cup	100	10	2½ Vegetable ½ Fat
Oven French Fries	½ cup	100	5	2 Bread
Peppered Veal	2½ ounces	225	208	2½ Meat 1 Vegetable ½ Bread ½ Fat
Low-Sodium Peppered Veal	2½ ounces	225	50	2½ Meat 1 Vegetable ½ Bread ½ Fat
Pita Crackers	1 cracker	10	23	⅛ Bread
Ricotta-Parmesan Torte	1 piece	250	365	1½ Bread 1 Meat ½ Vegetable 1 Fat
Seafood Quiche	⅛ pie	184	475	2½ Meat ½ Milk
Low-Sodium Seafood Quiche	⅛ pie	169	350	2½ Meat ½ Milk
Shishkabob	3 ounces	257	295	3 Meat 2 Vegetable
Shrimp Creole	1¾ cup	282	450	2 Meat 1½ Bread 2 Vegetable

Recipes	Amount	Calories	Sodium (mg)	Exchanges
Low-Sodium Shrimp Creole	1¾ cup	282	291	2 Meat 1½ Bread 2 Vegetable
Southern Fried Chicken	⅙ recipe	262	260	4 Meat ½ Bread ½ Fat
Low-Sodium Southern Fried Chicken	⅙ recipe	262	98	4 Meat ½ Bread ½ Fat
Spanish Chicken and Rice	1 cup	421	375	3½ Meat 2 Bread 1 Fat 2 Vegetable
Spicy Bean Enchiladas	1 piece	200	553	1 Meat 2 Bread ½ Vegetable
Low-Sodium Spicy Bean Enchiladas	1 piece	200	354	1 Meat 2 Bread ½ Vegetable
Spicy Tomato Sauce	4 tablespoons	28	340	1 Vegetable
Stuffed Shells	3 shells	320	150	2 Bread 3 Vegetable 1 Meat ½ Fat
Teriyaki Steak	4 ounces	280	472	4 Meat ½ Fat ½ Vegetable
Tuna Salad	½ cup	190	707	2 Meat 1 Milk
Low-Sodium Tuna Salad	½ cup	190	225	2 Meat 1 Milk
Turkey Fruit Salad	1 cup	185	150	1½ Meat 2 Fruit 1 Vegetable
Veal Scaloppine	3 ounces	290	252	3 Meat 1½ Vegetable 1 Fat 1 Bread
Vegetarian Lasagna	⅛ recipe	350	350	2 Bread 2 Meat 2½ Vegetable ½ Fat

III

Nutritional Contents of Fast Foods

Fast Foods

	Calories	Fat (gm)	Chol* (mg)	Sodium (mg)	% Fat
Arby's					
Junior Roast Beef	218	9	20	345	37
Regular Roast Beef	353	15	39	588	38
Giant Roast Beef	531	23	65	908	39
Philly Beef'N Swiss	460	28	107	1300	55
King Roast Beef	467	19	49	766	37
Super Roast Beef	501	22	40	798	40
Beef'N Cheddar	455	27	63	955	53
Bac'N Cheddar Deluxe	526	37	83	1672	63
Chicken Breast Sandwich	509	29	83	1082	51
Turkey Deluxe	375	17	39	1047	41
Hot Ham'N Cheese	292	14	45	1350	43
Fish Fillet Sandwich	580	32	70	928	50
Potato Cakes	201	13	13	397	58
Burger King					
Whopper Sandwich	628	36	90	880	52
w/cheese	711	43	113	1164	54
Bacon Double Cheeseburger	510	31	104	728	55
Whopper Junior Sandwich	322	17	41	486	48
w/cheese	364	20	52	628	49
Hamburger	275	12	37	509	39
Cheeseburger	317	15	48	651	43
Ham & Cheese Sandwich	471	23	70	1534	44
Chicken Sandwich	688	40	82	1423	52
Chicken Tenders (6 pcs.)	204	10	47	636	44
Whaler Fish Sandwich	488	27	77	592	50
Garden Salad	110	6	10	170	49
Side Salad	20	0	0	10	0
Chef Salad	180	11	120	610	55
Chunky Chicken Salad	140	4	50	440	26
Breakfast Croissan'wich	304	19	243	637	56
w/bacon	355	24	248	762	61
w/sausage	538	41	293	1042	69
w/ham	335	20	262	987	54

* Chol = Cholesterol

	Calories	Fat (gm)	Chol* (mg)	Sodium (mg)	% Fat
(cont'd)					
Bagel, Egg & Cheese					
w/bacon	438	19	273	905	39
w/ham	418	15	286	1130	32
w/sausage	621	36	317	1185	52
Scrambled Egg Platter	468	30	370	808	58
w/sausage	700	52	420	1213	67
w/bacon	536	58	378	975	97
French Toast Sticks	499	29	74	498	52
Great Danish	500	36	6	288	65
Cookies & Cream Spooners	270	10	N.A.	210	33
Church's Fried Chicken					
Breast	278	17	N.A.	560	55
Wing Breast	303	20	N.A.	583	59
Thigh	306	22	N.A.	448	65
Leg	147	9	N.A.	286	55
Corn-on-the-Cob, buttered	237	9	N.A.	20	34
Dairy Queen					
Single Hamburger	360	16	45	630	40
w/cheese	410	20	50	790	44
Double Hamburger	530	28	85	660	48
w/cheese	650	37	95	980	51
Chicken Sandwich	640	41	75	870	58
Fish Sandwich	400	17	50	875	38
w/cheese	440	21	60	1035	43
Hot Dog	280	16	45	830	51
w/chili	320	20	55	985	56
w/cheese	330	21	55	990	57
Super Hot Dog	520	27	80	1365	47
w/chili	570	32	100	1595	51
w/cheese	580	34	100	1605	53
DQ Dip Cone, small	190	9	10	55	42
regular	340	16	20	100	42
large	510	24	30	145	42
DQ Banana Split	540	11	30	150	18
Hot Fudge Brownie Delight	600	25	20	225	38

* Chol = Cholesterol
  N.A. = Not Available

	Calories	Fat (gm)	Chol* (mg)	Sodium (mg)	% Fat
Jack in the Box					
Hamburger	267	11	26	556	37
Cheeseburger	315	14	41	746	40
Double Cheeseburger	467	27	72	842	52
Jumbo Jack	584	34	73	733	52
Jumbo Jack w/cheese	677	40	102	1090	53
Bacon Cheeseburger	705	39	85	1127	50
Swiss & Bacon Burger	678	47	92	1458	62
Ultimate Cheeseburger	942	69	127	1176	66
Chicken Supreme	575	36	62	1525	56
Grilled Chicken Sandwich	447	19	N.A.	845	38
Chicken Strips (6 pcs.)	523	20	103	1122	34
Fish Supreme	554	32	66	1047	52
Shrimp (10 pcs.)	270	16	84	669	53
Beef Fajita Pita	333	14	45	635	38
Chicken Fajita Pita	292	8	34	703	25
Club Pita w/o sauce	277	8	43	931	26
Hot Club Supreme	524	28	82	1467	48
Taco	191	11	21	406	51
Super Taco	288	17	37	765	53
Guacamole	55	5	0	130	81
Egg Rolls (3 pcs.)	405	19	30	903	42
Chef Salad	325	18	142	900	50
Mexican Chicken Salad	443	21	104	1530	43
Taco Salad	641	38	91	1670	53
Side Salad	51	3	4	84	53
Supreme Crescent	547	40	178	1053	66
Sausage Crescent	584	43	187	1012	66
Canadian Crescent	452	31	226	851	62
Breakfast Jack	307	13	203	871	38
Scrambled Egg Platter	662	40	354	1188	54
Hash Browns	116	7	3	211	54
Pancake Platter	612	22	99	888	32
Cheesecake	309	18	63	208	52

* Chol = Cholesterol
  N.A. = Not Available

	Calories	Fat (gm)	Chol* (mg)	Sodium (mg)	% Fat
Kentucky Fried Chicken					
Original Recipe Chicken					
Wing	118	12	67	387	92
Side Breast	276	17	96	654	55
Center Breast	257	14	93	532	49
Drumstick	147	9	81	269	55
Thigh	278	19	122	517	62
Extra Crispy Chicken					
Wing	218	16	63	437	66
Side Breast	354	24	66	797	61
Center Breast	353	21	93	842	54
Drumstick	173	11	65	346	57
Thigh	371	26	121	766	63
Kentucky Nuggets (6 pcs.)	276	17	71	840	55
Mashed Potatoes	59	.5	0	228	8
Mashed Potatoes w/gravy	62	1	0	297	15
Chicken Gravy	59	4	2	398	61
Corn-on-the-Cob	176	3	0	10	15
Cole Slaw	103	6	4	171	52
Potato Salad	141	9	11	396	57
Baked Beans	105	1	0	387	9
Buttermilk Biscuit	269	14	0	521	47
Long John Silver's					
Chicken Planks (4 pcs.)	440	24	60	1280	49
Fish w/batter (2 pcs.)	300	16	60	1020	48
Catfish Fillet (2 pcs.)	400	24	60	700	54
Breaded Shrimp (1 order)	190	10	40	470	47
Battered Shrimp (6 pcs.)	240	18	60	720	68
Breaded Clams	240	12	<5	410	45
Crispy Breaded Fish Sandwich	600	28	30	1220	42
Clam Chowder w/cod (7 oz.)	140	6	20	590	39
Gumbo (7 oz.)	120	8	25	740	60
Seafood Salad w/2 crackers	270	7	90	660	23
Ocean Chef Salad w/2 crackers	250	9	80	1340	32
Cole Slaw	140	6	15	260	39

* Chol = Cholesterol

	Calories	Fat (gm)	Chol* (mg)	Sodium (mg)	% Fat
(cont'd)					
Mixed Vegetables	60	2	0	330	30
Corn-on-the-Cob, buttered	270	14	<5	95	47
Hushpuppies (3 pcs.)	210	6	<5	75	26
Pecan Pie (1 slice)	530	25	70	470	42
Lemon Meringue Pie (1 slice)	260	7	<5	270	24

McDonald's

	Calories	Fat (gm)	Chol* (mg)	Sodium (mg)	% Fat
Hamburger	263	11	29	506	38
Cheeseburger	318	16	41	743	45
Quarter Pounder	427	24	81	718	51
w/cheese	525	32	107	1220	55
Big Mac	570	35	83	979	55
McD.L.T.	680	44	101	1030	58
Chicken McNuggets (6 pcs.)	323	21	73	512	59
Filet-O-Fish	435	26	45	799	54
Chef Salad	226	13	125	850	52
Shrimp Salad	99	3	187	570	27
Garden Salad	91	6	110	100	59
Chicken Salad Oriental	146	4	92	270	25
Side Salad	48	3	42	45	56
Egg McMuffin	340	16	259	885	42
Sausage McMuffin	427	26	59	942	55
w/egg	517	33	287	1044	57
Biscuit, Plain	330	18	9	786	49
w/sausage	467	31	48	1147	60
w/sausage & egg	585	40	285	1301	62
w/bacon, egg & cheese	483	32	263	1269	60
Scrambled Eggs	180	13	514	205	65
Hot Cakes w/butter & syrup	500	10	47	1070	18
Sausage	210	19	39	423	81
Hash Brown Potatoes	125	7	7	325	50
English Muffin w/butter	186	5	15	310	24
Soft Serve Cone	185	5	24	109	24
Sundae, all flavors	346	10	28	135	26
McDonaldland Cookies	308	11	10	358	32
Chocolaty Chip Cookies	342	16	18	313	42

* Chol = Cholesterol

	Calories	Fat (gm)	Chol* (mg)	Sodium (mg)	% Fat
Pizza Hut					
(serving size—2 slices of medium 13-inch pizza; 4 servings per pizza)					
Thin'n Crispy					
Standard Cheese	340	11	22	900	29
Superstyle Cheese	410	14	30	1100	31
Standard Pepperoni	370	15	27	1000	36
Superstyle Pepperoni	430	19	34	1200	40
Standard Pork w/mushroom	380	14	35	1200	33
Superstyle Pork w/mushroom	450	19	40	1400	38
Supreme	400	17	13	1200	38
Super Supreme	520	26	44	1500	45
Thick'n Chewy					
Standard Cheese	390	10	18	800	23
Superstyle Cheese	450	14	21	1000	28
Standard Pepperoni	450	16	21	900	32
Superstyle Pepperoni	490	20	24	1200	37
Standard Pork w/mushroom	430	14	21	1000	29
Superstyle Pork w/mushroom	500	18	21	1200	32
Supreme	480	18	24	1000	34
Super Supreme	590	26	38	1400	40
Taco Bell					
Bean Burrito	360	11	14	922	28
Beef Burrito	402	17	59	994	38
Burrito Supreme	422	19	35	952	41
Double Beef Burrito Supreme	465	23	59	1054	45
Tostada	243	11	18	670	41
Enchirito	382	20	56	1260	47
Mexican Pizza	714	48	81	1364	61
Pintos & Cheese	194	9	19	733	42
Nachos	356	19	9	423	48
Nachos Bellgrande	720	41	43	1312	51

* Chol = Cholesterol

	Calories	Fat (gm)	Chol* (mg)	Sodium (mg)	% Fat
(cont'd)					
Taco	184	11	32	273	54
Taco Bellgrande	351	22	55	470	56
Taco Light	412	29	57	575	63
Soft Taco	229	12	32	516	47
Taco Salad w/salsa	949	62	85	1763	59
Taco Salad w/o shell	525	32	82	1522	55
Fajita Steak Taco	236	11	14	507	42
Chicken Fajita	225	N.A.	N.A.	N.A.	N.A.
Maxi Melt	264	N.A.	N.A.	N.A.	N.A.
Cinnamon Crispas	266	16	2	122	54
Cheesearito	312	13	29	451	38

Wendy's

	Calories	Fat (gm)	Chol* (mg)	Sodium (mg)	% Fat
Hamburger	260	9	30	510	31
Cheeseburger	320	15	50	805	42
†Single Hamburger	430	22	70	805	46
w/cheese	490	28	85	1100	51
†Double Hamburger	640	36	145	910	51
w/cheese	700	42	160	1205	54
†Triple Hamburger	850	50	220	1015	50
w/cheese	970	62	250	1605	58
†Bacon Cheeseburger	535	31	78	993	52
Philly Swiss Burger	510	24	65	975	42
†Bacon Swiss Burger	710	44	90	1390	56
†Wendy's Big Classic w/cheese	640	40	100	1310	56
Chicken Breast Fillet	200	10	60	310	45
†Chicken Sandwich	430	19	60	705	40
Crispy Chicken Nuggets (6 pcs.)	310	21	50	660	61
Chili	230	9	50	960	35
Hot Stuffed Baked Potatoes					
Plain (9 oz.)	250	2	0	60	7
Sour Cream/Chives	460	24	15	230	47
Cheese	590	34	22	450	52
Chili & Cheese	510	20	22	610	35
Bacon & Cheese	570	30	22	1180	47
Broccoli & Cheese	500	25	22	430	45

* Chol = Cholesterol
  N.A. = Not Available
† Includes mayonnaise

	Calories	Fat (gm)	Chol* (mg)	Sodium (mg)	% Fat
(cont'd)					
Garden Salad (take-out)	102	5	0	110	44
Chef Salad (take-out)	180	9	120	140	45
Taco Salad	660	37	35	1110	50
Delux Three Bean Salad (¼ cup)	60	0	N.A.	15	0
Red Bliss Potato Salad (¼ cup)	110	9	N.A.	265	74
Pasta Deli Salad (¼ cup)	35	0	N.A.	120	0
California Cole Slaw (¼ cup)	60	6	10	140	90
Turkey Ham (¼ cup)	50	2	N.A.	N.A.	36
Taco Shell (1)	50	2	N.A.	0	36
Flour Tortilla	110	3	N.A.	220	25
Taco Chips (2 oz.)	260	10	N.A.	20	35
Fettucini (1 cup)	296	7	0	7	21
Rotini (1 cup)	226	5	0	0	18
Pasta Medley (1 cup)	156	5	0	7	29
Alfredo Sauce (½ cup)	110	4	N.A.	44	33
Spaghetti Sauce (½ cup)	88	0	0	872	0
Cheese Sauce (½ cup)	110	4	N.A.	916	33
Frosty (small)	400	14	50	220	32
Pudding, all flavors (½ cup)	180	8	0	156	80

Miscellaneous

Beverages (8 oz.)

	Calories	Fat (gm)	Chol* (mg)	Sodium (mg)	% Fat
Coffee	3	0	0	2	0
Tea	3	0	0	0	0
Orange Juice (6 oz.)	85	0	0	2	0
Chocolate Milk, Low-fat	180	5	5	150	25
Skim Milk	90	.4	5	125	0
2% Milk	140	5	5	145	32
Whole Milk	155	9	34	120	52
Soft Drink (12 oz.)	167	0	0	30	0
Diet Soft Drink (12 oz.)	1	0	0	58	0
Milkshake, vanilla	338	9	22	244	24
Milkshake, chocolate	398	11	36	276	25

* Chol = Cholesterol
  N.A. = Not Available

	Calories	Fat (gm)	Chol* (mg)	Sodium (mg)	% Fat
(cont'd)					
Extras					
Catsup (2 Tbsp.)	30	0	0	310	0
Jelly (1 Tbsp.)	55	0	0	2	0
Table Syrup (2 Tbsp.)	100	0	0	4	0
Coffeemate (1 pkt.)	17	1	0	6	53
†Dressings (1 Tbsp.)					
Lemon Juice or Vinegar	0	0	0	0	0
Blue Cheese	75	8	4	165	96
French	65	6	1	220	83
Italian	85	9	1	315	95
Thousand Island	80	8	8	110	90
Ranch	53	5.5	4	186	94
Oil & Vinegar	72	8	0	.1	100
Low-calorie Dressings (Avg.)	18	1	2	144	50
French Fries, regular order	221	11	10	120	41
large order	353	19	13	262	48
jumbo order	442	24	16	328	49
Onion Rings	328	20	27	536	55
Fried Pie	316	17	11	341	48
Tartar Sauce (1 pkt.)	80	3	5	80	34
Sweet & Sour Sauce (1 pkt.)	40	0	0	160	0
BBQ Sauce (1 pkt.)	44	N.A.	N.A.	300	N.A.
Cocktail Sauce (1 pkt.)	32	0	0	206	0
Picante Sauce (1 Tbsp.)	7	0	0	74	0

* Chol = Cholesterol

N.A. = Not Available

† check packet to determine serving size

IV

Calorie, Fat, Cholesterol, and Sodium Content of Commonly Used Foods

Food	Amount	Kcal	Fat (gm)	Chol (mg)	Sodium (mg)
Apple, fresh	1 medium	80	0	0	1
juice	½ cup	60	0	0	1
Applesauce, canned,					
sweetened	½ cup	105	0	0	3
unsweetened	½ cup	50	0	0	2
Apricots, fresh	3 small	50	0	0	1
canned, sweetened	½ cup (4 halves)	100	0	0	1
dried	¼ cup (4 halves)	80	0	0	9
nectar	½ cup	70	0	0	0
Asparagus, fresh	½ cup	20	0	0	1
canned	½ cup	20	0	0	235
Avocado, fresh	½ medium	190	18	0	5
dip (guacamole)	½ cup	140	13	0	165
Banana, fresh	1 6-inch long	100	0	0	1
Bacon, cooked	2 slices	109	10	16	303
bits	1 tablespoon	36	2	0	432
Canadian	1 slice	65	4	10	442
Baking powder	1 teaspoon	4	0	0	405
Baking soda	1 teaspoon	0	0	0	821
Bean dip	1 tablespoon	20	1	2	177
Bean sprouts	1 cup	35	0	0	5
Beans	½ cup	118	0	0	7
baked	½ cup	190	6	0	485
garbanzo, cooked	½ cup	134	2	0	6
green, cooked	½ cup	15	0	0	2
kidney, canned	½ cup	112	0	0	4
navy, cooked	½ cup	88	0	0	0
pinto, cooked	½ cup	92	0	0	0
pork and beans,					
cooked	½ cup	160	4	1	59
refried beans	½ cup	230	12	0	340
Beef, barbecued					
sandwich with bun	1 sandwich	509	37	81	506
brisket, baked	3 ounces	367	33	80	46
barbecued	3 ounces	382	34	80	176
chicken fried					
steak	4 ounces	370	22	130	350
chop suey	1 cup	300	17	64	1052
chuck roast,					
baked	3 ounces	240	17	60	40
corned beef	3 ounces	372	30	83	1740
flank steak	3 ounces	158	5	50	47

Food	Amount	Kcal	Fat (gm)	Chol (mg)	Sodium (mg)
(Beef-continued)					
hamburger					
patty, broiled	3 ounces	190	10	50	60
jerky	1 piece	38	2	10	418
liver, fried	3 ounces	200	9	255	155
meatloaf	3 ounces	171	11	50	555
paté	1 tablespoon	41	14	40	91
pot pie	1 piece	443	24	41	1008
prime rib, baked	3 ounces	380	33	80	40
round steak	3 ounces	220	13	60	60
short ribs	1 rib	290	24	24	39
sirloin steak,					
broiled	3 ounces	330	27	80	50
stew	1 cup	220	11	63	90
stroganoff	1 cup	470	33	130	860
sweetbreads	3 ounces	143	3	466	0
tenderloin (fillet)	3 ounces	174	8	72	54
Beet greens, cooked	½ cup	15	0	0	55
Beets, canned	½ cup	30	0	0	200
Beverages, beer	12 ounces	150	0	0	25
beer, non-alcoholic	12 ounces	65	0	0	0
club soda	6 ounces	0	0	0	30
coffee	1 cup	3	0	0	2
Gatorade	1 cup	39	0	0	123
ginger ale	12 ounces	105	0	0	4
Kool Aid	1 cup	100	0	0	1
lemonade	1 cup	110	0	0	1
mineral water	1 cup	0	0	0	5
quinine water	1 cup	74	0	0	16
soft drinks, all					
canned	12 ounces	150	0	0	10–30
Tang	1 cup	135	0	0	17
tea	1 cup	3	0	0	0
tonic water	12 ounces	132	0	0	0
V-8 juice	6 ounces	31	0	0	364
whiskey	1½ ounces	107	0	0	0
wine	4 ounces	85	0	0	5
Blackberries, fresh	1 cup	80	0	0	2
Blackeyed peas,					
canned	¾ cup	81	0	0	602
dried, cooked	1 cup	72	1	0	2
Blueberries, fresh	1 cup	90	0	0	2
Bouillon cube	1 cube	18	1	0	960
low-sodium	1 cube	18	1	0	10

Food	Amount	Kcal	Fat (gm)	Chol (mg)	Sodium (mg)
Bread, bagel	1 piece	180	2	0	260
biscuit	1 piece	90	3	2	270
diet	1 slice	40	0	0	115
breadstick	1 piece	23	0	0	100
cornbread	1 piece	180	6	3	265
cornbread muffin	1 2-inch muffin	130	4	2	190
croissant	1 piece	180	11	48	270
croutons	2 cups	359	1	0	1360
English muffin	1 muffin	138	1	0	203
French bread	1 slice	70	0	0	145
mixed grain bread	1 slice	64	1	0	103
pita pocket	1 pita	170	2	0	53
popover	1 medium	112	5	74	110
raisin bread	1 slice	65	0	1	90
roll, dinner	1 small	85	2	1	140
hard	1 small	160	2	0	315
whole wheat	1 small	90	1	0	197
rye bread	1 slice	65	0	1	140
sweet roll	1 medium	270	16	46	240
white bread	1 slice	70	0	1	130
whole wheat bread	1 slice	65	0	1	130
Broccoli, cooked	½ cup	20	0	0	8
raw	1 cup	24	0	0	24
Brussels sprouts	½ cup	30	0	0	8
Butter, regular	1 teaspoon	35	4	13	40
unsalted	1 teaspoon	36	4	11	0
Cabbage, cooked	½ cup	15	0	0	10
Cake (1 piece), angel food	¹⁄₁₂ cake	135	0	0	60
brownie without icing	2-inch x 2-inch	146	10	25	75
cheese cake, plain	¹⁄₁₂ cake	255	13	60	170
chocolate cake with icing	¹⁄₁₂ cake	379	16	62	322
cupcake with icing	1 cupcake	190	6	54	160
fruitcake	¹⁄₃₀ cake	55	2	0	21
gingerbread	2-inch x 2-inch	170	5	0	190
pound cake	¹⁄₁₇ cake	140	9	48	35
Candy, caramels	3 pieces	120	3	2	65
chocolate chips	2 tablespoons	148	8	2	64
fudge	1 ounce	120	5	5	50

Food	Amount	Kcal	Fat (gm)	Chol (mg)	Sodium (mg)
(Candy-continued)					
gum	1 piece	9	0	0	0
gum drop, small	2 tablespoons	100	0	25	10
hard candy	1 ounce	110	0	0	10
jelly beans	¼ cup	66	0	0	0
milk chocolate	1.65 ounces	140	9	4	25
peanut brittle	1 ounce	120	3	2	10
peanut butter cup	1 piece	130	8	1	75
Cantaloupe	¼ melon	50	0	0	20
Carrots, cooked	½ cup	20	0	0	25
Cauliflower, cooked	½ cup	15	0	0	10
Celery, raw	1 stalk	15	0	0	100
Cereals, All Bran	1 cup	210	2	0	960
Alpha Bits	1 cup	119	0	0	227
bran	1 cup	120	2	0	60
Bran Buds	1 cup	210	2	0	516
bran flakes	1 cup	127	0	0	363
Cheerios	1 cup	89	1	0	297
corn flakes	1 cup	95	0	0	325
Cream of Wheat, cooked	½ cup	50	0	0	175
granola	1 cup	503	20	0	232
Grape Nuts	1 cup	402	0	0	299
Malt-O-Meal, cooked	½ cup	61	0	0	1
oat bran, dry	⅓ cup	110	2	0	0
oatmeal, cooked	½ cup	69	1	0	218
Product 19	1 cup	126	0	0	386
Puffed Rice	1 cup	54	0	0	1
Puffed Wheat	1 cup	50	0	0	1
Raisin Bran	1 cup	155	1	0	293
Ralston, cooked	½ cup	67	0	0	2
Rice Chex	1 cup	110	0	0	240
Rice Krispies	1 cup	112	0	0	340
Shredded Wheat	1 cup	180	1	0	2
Special K	1 cup	76	0	0	154
Sugar Crisp	1 cup	121	0	0	29
Sugar Pops	1 cup	109	0	0	103
Team flakes	1 cup	109	1	0	175
Total	1 cup	109	1	0	352
wheat flakes	1 cup	100	0	0	310
wheat germ	⅓ cup	120	4	0	0
Cheese, American	1 ounce	110	9	50	405
blue cheese	1 ounce	100	8	21	395

Food	Amount	Kcal	Fat (gm)	Chol (mg)	Sodium (mg)
(Cheese-continued)					
Brie	1 ounce	95	8	28	178
Camembert	1 ounce	85	7	20	239
cheddar	1 ounce	115	10	28	175
colby	1 ounce	112	9	27	171
cottage cheese,					
regular	½ cup	120	5	24	455
low-fat	½ cup	81	1	12	459
cream cheese	2 tablespoons	100	10	32	85
Edam	1 ounce	101	7	25	274
feta	1 ounce	75	6	25	316
Gouda	1 ounce	101	8	32	232
gruyere	1 ounce	117	9	31	95
low-calorie cheese	1 ounce	52	2	5	606
low-cholesterol					
cheese	1 ounce	110	9	5	150
Monterey jack	1 ounce	106	9	26	152
mozzarella, part-					
skim	1 ounce	72	5	16	132
muenster	1 ounce	104	9	27	178
Neufchâtel	1 ounce	74	6	22	113
Parmesan	⅓ cup	130	9	28	247
pimiento	¼ cup	106	9	27	405
provolone	1 ounce	100	8	20	248
ricotta cheese,					
regular	½ cup	216	16	63	104
part-skim	½ cup	170	10	38	153
Roquefort	1 ounce	100	8	45	395
Swiss	1 ounce	110	8	35	75
Cherries, fresh	½ cup	45	0	0	1
Chicken, breast, baked					
without skin	3 ounces	190	7	89	86
breast, fried	3 ounces	327	23	89	498
canned	½ cup	200	12	91	42
chow mein	1 cup	95	2	15	725
pot pie	1 piece	503	25	13	863
salad	½ cup	127	8	28	345
Chili, beef and bean	1 cup	340	15	34	1355
Chow mein noodles	½ cup	200	8	0	320
Cocoa powder	1 tablespoon	18	0	0	25
Coconut	4 tablespoons	180	12	0	7

Food	Amount	Kcal	Fat (gm)	Chol (mg)	Sodium (mg)
Coffee creamer, non-dairy					
liquid	1 tablespoon	20	2	0	12
powder	1 teaspoon	11	1	0	4
Cole slaw	1 cup	118	8	7	149
Cookies, animal					
crackers	5	43	1	4	30
chocolate chip	1	57	8	2	64
Fig Newton	1	50	1	17	35
ginger snaps	3	50	1	0	69
graham cracker	1	55	1	8	95
molasses cookie	1	71	3	7	58
oatmeal cookie	1	80	3	7	69
Oreo cookie	1	49	2	0	63
peanut butter cookie	1	232	10	0	85
Rice Krispie bar	2-inch x 2-inch	225	10	0	80
shortbread cookie	1	42	2	0	36
sugar cookie	1	98	3	0	109
vanilla wafers	3	51	2	9	28
Cool Whip	1 tablespoon	14	1	0	1
Corn, on-the-cob	1 ear	169	1	0	0
canned	½ cup	70	1	0	195
creamed, canned	½ cup	110	1	0	300
frozen	½ cup	70	0	0	0
Crackers (see Snack foods)					
Cranberry, fresh	1 cup	46	0	0	0
juice	¾ cup	106	0	0	0
Cream, half and half	1 tablespoon	20	2	6	6
heavy	1 tablespoon	52	6	24	6
sour	1 tablespoon	26	3	5	6
whipped	½ cup	210	22	80	20
whipping cream, heavy	1 tablespoon	52	6	21	6
light	1 tablespoon	44	5	17	5
Cucumber	½ cup	10	0	0	4
Custard	½ cup	150	8	139	105
Dates	½ cup	220	0	0	1
Donuts, cake	1	160	8	33	210
glazed	1	180	11	16	100
Egg	1	80	6	252	60
Egg substitute	¼ cup	25	0	0	80

Food	Amount	Kcal	Fat (gm)	Chol (mg)	Sodium (mg)
Egg noodles, cooked	1 cup	220	3	55	15
Figs, fresh	1 piece	80	0	0	2
dried	2 pieces	274	1	0	34
Fish, bass, baked	3 ounces	82	2	68	59
caviar	1 tablespoon	42	2	94	352
cod, baked	3 ounces	180	6	56	115
crab	3 ounces	100	2	100	850
fish sticks	4	200	10	70	115
flounder, baked	3 ounces	200	8	51	235
haddock, baked	3 ounces	180	7	66	195
halibut, baked	3 ounces	175	4	51	86
herring, canned	½ cup	208	11	85	74
lobster	3 ounces	90	2	85	205
mackerel, baked	3 ounces	250	17	95	35
mussels	¼ cup	48	1	16	104
oysters, fresh	6	80	2	60	90
fried	6	138	8	131	116
perch	3 ounces	227	13	55	153
pike	3 ounces	116	2	55	64
red snapper	3 ounces	93	1	55	67
salmon, baked with butter	3 ounces	189	12	58	116
canned in water	½ cup	160	6	75	425
patty, fried	3 ounces	239	12	64	96
smoked	3 ounces	150	8	85	425
sardines	¼ cup	58	3	28	184
scallops	3 ounces	105	2	53	250
shrimp, boiled	1 cup	100	1	119	250
fried	1 cup	380	19	240	320
sole, baked	3 ounces	141	1	51	235
sushi (raw fish)	3 ounces	93	1	50	67
swordfish, baked	3 ounces	174	6	43	98
trout	3 ounces	196	5	55	61
tuna, canned in oil	3 ounces	176	9	19	535
canned in water	3 ounces	109	2	30	399
canned in water, low-sodium	3 ounces	106	2	30	33
steak	3 ounces	145	4	60	0
Frankfurter	1	261	17	45	776
Fruit cocktail, canned, sweetened	½ cup	95	0	0	5
Grapefruit, fresh	½ medium	40	0	0	1
juice, unsweetened	1 cup	93	0	0	3

Food	Amount	Kcal	Fat (gm)	Chol (mg)	Sodium (mg)
Grapes, fresh	1 cup	70	0	0	4
juice	¾ cup	120	0	0	4
Green chiles, canned	1 tablespoon	14	0	0	0
Green pepper, raw	½ cup	15	0	0	10
Greens, collard, cooked	⅓ cup	20	0	0	35
kale, cooked	1 cup	41	0	0	30
spinach, cooked	½ cup	20	0	0	50
spinach, raw	½ cup	7	0	0	19
Swiss chard, cooked	½ cup	15	0	0	60
turnip, cooked	½ cup	15	0	0	19
Grits, cooked	½ cup	73	0	0	0
Ham, baked, lean	3 ounces	203	8	74	1684
Honey	1 tablespoon	65	0	0	1
Honeydew	¼ melon	55	0	0	20
Ice cream, regular (10 percent fat)	½ cup	135	7	36	60
rich (16 percent fat)	½ cup	266	14	72	120
soft serve	½ cup	163	10	0	51
Ice milk	½ cup	90	3	13	50
Instant breakfast	1 cup	280	8	28	242
Jalapeno pepper, canned	¼ cup	132	0	0	497
Jam or jelly	1 tablespoon	55	0	0	2
Jello	½ cup	70	0	0	0
Kiwi	1 piece	46	0	0	4
Knockwurst	3 ounces	278	23	65	483
Lamb chop, baked	3 ounces	340	28	85	50
roast, baked	3 ounces	160	6	59	60
Lasagna	1 cup	380	12	67	43
Lemon, fresh	¼ lemon	22	0	0	3
juice	1 tablespoon	5	0	0	0
Lentils	⅔ cup	110	0	0	10
Lettuce	1 cup	6	0	0	6
Lima beans	½ cup	95	0	0	2
Lime, fresh	¼ lime	20	0	0	1
juice	1 tablespoon	3	0	0	2
Luncheon meats, bologna	1 ounce	85	8	28	370
pepperoni	1 ounce	139	13	70	492
pimiento loaf	1 ounce	74	6	10	394
salami	1 ounce	130	11	15	350

Food	Amount	Kcal	Fat (gm)	Chol (mg)	Sodium (mg)
Macaroni and cheese	1 cup	430	22	42	1085
Macaroni, cooked	1 cup	210	1	0	0
Mandarin oranges, canned	½ cup	76	0	0	8
Mango	1 cup	110	0	0	10
Margarine, low-calorie	1 teaspoon	16	2	0	49
regular	1 teaspoon	35	4	0	50
unsalted	1 teaspoon	35	4	0	0
Marshmallows	½ cup	90	0	0	10
Milk, buttermilk, skim	1 cup	90	0	5	318
chocolate, low-fat	1 cup	180	5	5	150
evaporated milk, regular	1 cup	340	20	77	265
evaporated milk, skimmed	1 cup	199	0	10	293
hot chocolate	1 cup	110	3	35	154
low-fat (1 percent fat)	1 cup	102	3	3	122
low-fat (2 percent fat)	1 cup	140	5	5	145
nonfat (dry)	¼ cup	109	0	6	161
skim	1 cup	90	0	5	125
whole (4 percent fat)	1 cup	155	9	34	120
Mixed vegetables, canned	½ cup	38	0	0	121
frozen	½ cup	54	0	0	45
stir-fried	½ cup	59	5	0	17
Mushrooms, canned	⅓ cup	17	0	0	400
fresh	½ cup	10	0	0	5
Nectarine, fresh	1	64	0	0	6
Nuts and seeds, almonds, unsalted	¼ cup	180	16	0	56
brazil nuts, unsalted	¼ cup	180	19	0	0
cashews, unsalted	¼ cup	320	26	0	120
macadamia nuts, unsalted	¼ cup	109	12	0	60
mixed nuts, unsalted	¼ cup	214	20	0	4
peanuts, salted	¼ cup	330	28	0	157
peanuts, unsalted	¼ cup	330	28	0	1
pecans, unsalted	¼ cup	200	20	0	0

Food	Amount	Kcal	Fat (gm)	Chol (mg)	Sodium (mg)
(Nuts and seeds-continued)					
pistachio nuts, salted	¼ cup	88	8	0	60
sunflower seeds, unsalted	¼ cup	200	17	0	10
walnuts, unsalted	¼ cup	200	20	0	0
Okra, cooked	½ cup	30	0	0	2
Olives, black	5	35	4	0	150
green	5	20	3	0	465
Onion, green	1 tablespoon	1	0	0	0
Orange, fresh	1 medium	80	0	0	1
juice	¾ cup	85	0	0	2
Pancakes (4-inch diameter)	3 medium	210	2	63	600
Papaya	½ medium	60	0	0	4
Parsnips	½ cup	66	0	0	8
Peach, fresh	1 medium	40	0	0	1
canned, sweetened	⅔ cup	120	0	0	4
canned, unsweetened	⅔ cup	43	0	0	9
Peanut butter, regular	1 tablespoon	95	8	0	95
unsalted	1 tablespoon	95	9	0	5
Pear, fresh	1 medium	100	0	0	3
canned, sweetened	½ cup	65	0	0	2
canned, unsweetened	½ cup	35	0	0	3
Peas, canned	½ cup	75	0	0	200
frozen	½ cup	55	0	0	90
split	½ cup	115	0	0	15
Pickles, dill	1 large	15	0	0	1930
sweet	1 small	50	0	0	200
relish	1 tablespoon	20	0	0	105
Pie (1 slice), banana cream	⅛ pie	285	12	40	252
chocolate cream	⅛ pie	264	15	0	273
lemon meringue	⅛ pie	257	14	130	395
mincemeat	⅛ pie	365	16	0	604
pecan	⅛ pie	334	18	92	177
pumpkin	⅛ pie	320	17	150	325
rhubarb	⅛ pie	190	17	10	432
strawberry	⅛ pie	228	9	10	227
Pimientos, canned	¼ cup	11	0	0	0

Food	Amount	Kcal	Fat (gm)	Chol (mg)	Sodium (mg)
Pineapple, fresh	1 cup	80	0	0	2
canned, sweetened	1 cup	190	0	0	4
canned, unsweetened	1 cup	150	0	0	4
Pizza, cheese (13-inch diameter)	2 slices	340	11	2	900
combination (13-inch diameter)	2 slices	400	17	13	1200
pepperoni (13-inch diameter)	2 slices	370	15	27	1000
Plum, fresh	1 large	30	0	0	1
canned, sweetened	½ cup	110	0	0	1
canned, unsweetened	½ cup	51	0	0	1
Pork chop, broiled	3½ ounces	357	26	77	60
roast, baked	3 ounces	310	24	59	50
Potatoes, au gratin	½ cup	95	3	6	529
baked	1 medium	140	0	0	5
French fries	½ cup (10 pieces)	220	10	13	120
mashed	½ cup	100	5	15	350
tater tots	½ cup	200	12	20	545
Prunes, canned	1 cup	245	0	0	6
dried (5 pieces)	¼ cup	130	0	0	4
Pudding, banana	½ cup	241	6	25	11
chocolate	½ cup	167	5	65	160
low-calorie	½ cup	76	0	0	146
tapioca	½ cup	110	4	9	130
vanilla	½ cup	140	5	16	85
Quiche (1 slice), cheese	⅛ pie	448	39	305	869
cheese and bacon	⅛ pie	520	42	310	970
Radishes	½ cup	7	0	0	10
Raisins	¼ cup	100	0	0	10
Raspberries, fresh	½ cup	40	0	0	1
frozen	½ cup	128	0	0	0
Rhubarb, cooked, sweetened	½ cup	190	0	0	2
Rice, brown	⅔ cup	160	1	0	370
white	⅔ cup	150	0	0	2
wild	1 tablespoon	33	0	0	1
Rice-a-Roni	⅔ cup	165	5	13	820
Rice cake	1 cake	31	0	0	8

Food	Amount	Kcal	Fat (gm)	Chol (mg)	Sodium (mg)
Salad dressings					
blue cheese	1 tablespoon	75	8	4	165
blue cheese, low-calorie	1 tablespoon	10	1	4	177
French	1 tablespoon	65	6	1	220
French, low-calorie	1 tablespoon	22	0	1	128
green goddess	1 tablespoon	68	7	1	150
Italian	1 tablespoon	85	9	1	315
Italian, low-calorie	1 tablespoon	15	2	1	118
mayonnaise	1 tablespoon	100	11	8	85
mayonnaise, low-calorie	1 tablespoon	50	5	1	100
oil and vinegar	1 tablespoon	71	8	0	0
Ranch or buttermilk	1 tablespoon	53	5	4	185
Russian	1 tablespoon	76	8	0	133
thousand island	1 tablespoon	80	8	8	110
thousand island, low-calorie	1 tablespoon	24	2	2	153
Sauces and condiments					
barbecue	1 tablespoon	15	1	0	130
bearnaise	1 cup	701	68	189	1265
catsup	1 tablespoon	15	0	0	155
chili	1 tablespoon	17	0	0	228
chocolate	2 tablespoons	100	0	2	36
gravy	¼ cup	164	14	7	720
hollandaise	¼ cup	361	39	382	400
mustard	1 teaspoon	4	0	0	65
picante or salsa	1½ tablespoons	10	0	0	111
soy	2 tablespoons	25	0	0	2665
soy, low-sodium	2 tablespoons	25	0	0	1200
steak	1 tablespoon	18	0	0	149
tartar	2 tablespoons	75	8	10	100
teriyaki	1 tablespoon	15	0	0	690
white	½ cup	200	16	16	475
worcestershire	1 teaspoon	4	0	0	49
Sauerkraut	½ cup	20	0	0	880
Sausage, link	1	134	12	0	175
patty	1	112	8	34	418
Polish	3 ounces	276	24	60	744
Scallions	¼ cup	10	0	0	1
Shallots	⅓ cup	36	0	0	6
Sherbet	½ cup	134	1	0	10

Food	Amount	Kcal	Fat (gm)	Chol (mg)	Sodium (mg)
Snack foods and crackers					
Cheetos	1 cup	153	10	9	329
corn chips	1 cup	155	10	0	183
peanut butter cracker sandwich	1 sandwich	61	4	3	103
popcorn, air-popped	2 cups	80	1	0	0
popcorn, caramel	2 cups	270	2	0	0
popcorn, cheese	2 cups	130	8	5	280
popcorn, cooked with oil	2 cups	106	5	13	466
potato chips	1 cup	115	8	0	200
pretzels, sticks	50 sticks	109	1	0	875
pretzels, 3-ring	10 rings	120	2	0	500
rice cake	1 cake	31	0	0	8
Ritz crackers	5 crackers	76	3	8	180
Rykrisp crackers	2 crackers	40	0	0	110
saltines	4 squares	50	2	8	125
saltines, unsalted tops	4 squares	50	2	8	83
shoestring potato sticks	1 cup	152	10	3	280
tortilla chips	1 cup	135	6	0	99
trail mix	⅓ cup	189	10	0	236
Triscuit crackers	2 crackers	60	2	0	90
Wheat Thin crackers	4 crackers	70	3	0	120
Soups, bean	1 cup	170	6	10	1010
beef noodle	1 cup	84	3	5	952
black bean	1 cup	116	2	0	110
broth, beef	1 cup	16	0	0	782
broth, beef, low-sodium	1 cup	16	0	0	12
broth, chicken	1 cup	16	0	0	782
broth, chicken, low-sodium	1 cup	16	0	0	7
chicken noodle	1 cup	75	2	7	1107
cream of mushroom	1 cup	203	14	20	1076
gazpacho	1 cup	57	2	0	1183
gumbo, chicken	1 cup	200	4	22	970
lentil	1 cup	108	0	0	1038
minestrone	1 cup	83	3	2	911

Food	Amount	Kcal	Fat (gm)	Chol (mg)	Sodium (mg)
(Soups-continued)					
onion	1 cup	65	2	5	1051
onion, dehydrated	2 tablespoons	21	0	0	636
pea	1 cup	140	3	4	940
potato	1 cup	148	7	22	1060
tomato	1 cup	90	3	4	970
turkey	1 cup	136	4	9	923
vegetable	1 cup	78	4	0	1010
vegetable beef	1 cup	80	2	4	1050
vegetable, chunky	1 cup	122	4	0	1010
won ton	1 cup	92	2	1	2027
Spaghetti, cooked	1 cup	210	1	0	5
Spam	1 ounce	87	7	15	336
Squash (winter), baked	½ cup	65	0	0	1
Strawberries, fresh	⅔ cup	35	0	0	1
frozen, sweetened	⅔ cup	160	0	0	2
frozen, unsweetened	⅔ cup	119	0	0	2
Succotash	1 cup	222	2	0	32
Sweet potato or yam, baked	¾ cup	160	0	0	15
canned	¾ cup	216	5	10	67
Syrup, corn	1 tablespoon	58	0	0	14
maple	1 tablespoon	50	0	0	2
Taco shell	1 piece	135	6	0	99
Tangerine, fresh	1 medium	46	0	0	2
Tofu	½ cup	85	5	0	10
Tofutti	½ cup	230	14	0	95
Tomato, fresh	½ cup	25	0	0	4
canned, regular	½ cup	25	0	0	155
canned, no salt added	½ cup	25	0	0	20
juice	¾ cup	35	0	0	365
juice, low-sodium	¾ cup	31	0	0	18
paste	½ cup	110	1	0	50
sauce, canned	½ cup	43	0	0	656
sauce, canned, no salt added	½ cup	43	0	0	25
Tortilla, corn (6-inch diameter)	1	65	1	0	1
flour (8-inch diameter)	1	105	3	0	134

Food	Amount	Kcal	Fat (gm)	Chol (mg)	Sodium (mg)
Turkey, dark meat, baked without skin	3 ounces	170	7	64	85
light meat, baked without skin	3 ounces	150	4	64	70
roll, light and dark meat	3 ounces	126	6	48	498
turkey ham	3 ounces	73	3	0	563
Turnips	½ cup	20	0	0	25
Veal cutlet	3 ounces	231	13	76	55
patty	3 ounces	298	19	90	51
Waffle	4-inch square	124	5	32	340
Water chestnuts, canned	¼ cup	20	0	0	5
Watercress	1 cup	5	0	0	20
Watermelon	2 ¾ cup	110	0	0	5
Yogurt, plain, nonfat	1 cup	127	68	4	174
frozen	½ cup	108	1	0	0
Zucchini, cooked	1 cup	22	0	0	2
raw	1 cup	38	0	0	3